Psychopathology in Childhood

SOCIAL, DIAGNOSTIC, AND THERAPEUTIC ASPECTS

Mary Engel

City College of the City University of New York

UNDER THE GENERAL EDITORSHIP OF
Jerome Kagan, HARVARD UNIVERSITY

Harcourt Brace Jovanovich, Inc.
New York / Chicago / San Francisco / Atlanta

DEDICATED TO THE MEMORY OF
Helen D. Sargent
1904–1959

ISBN: 0-15-573028-2

Library of Congress Catalog Card Number: 73-190750

Printed in the United States of America

Acknowledgments

The author wishes to thank the companies listed below for permission to reprint material in this book.

Pp. 12, 13, 14: Excerpts from articles by Robert Reinhold, Robert E. Tomasson, and Juan M. Vasquez © 1970 by The New York Times Company. Reprinted by permission.

Pp. 69–71: Classification system reprinted by permission from pp. 217–19 of *Psychopathological Disorders in Childhood,* Group for the Advancement of Psychiatry, Committee on Child Psychiatry, 1966.

Pp. 119–123: Excerpts from *Neurotic Styles* by David Shapiro © 1965 by Hafner Publishing Company, Inc. Reprinted by permission.

Pp. 133–34: Excerpts from *The Collected Papers of Sigmund Freud,* Vol. III, Ernest Jones, ed., and Alix and James Strachey, trans., published by Basic Books, Inc., by arrangement with The Hogarth Press Ltd. and The Institute of Psycho-Analysis, London. Reprinted by permission of Basic Books, Inc., Sigmund Freud Copyrights Ltd., The Institute of Psycho-Analysis, and The Hogarth Press Ltd.

48949

Preface

The purpose of *Psychopathology in Childhood* is to acquaint the student with some facts, issues, and problems in child clinical psychology today. Selected topics are presented in the general framework of three foci: the social, diagnostic, and therapeutic aspects of mental illness in children. The choice of topics for detailed discussion was guided by my judgment and experience as a teacher. Highest priority was given to those topics that assume no prior preparation in any of the subspecialties of psychology and that are most likely to involve young people in the future of those even younger.

Thus, the book is intended primarily as a companion volume to general textbooks in the areas of child health, mental health, and child development. It can be used as a supplement in undergraduate courses in abnormal psychology, child psychology, psychopathology, and education. An extensive list of suggested readings at the end of the book directs the student to topics that are not discussed or that are of necessity touched on only briefly in the text.

The structure of the book reflects the belief that social attitudes and public policy are the backdrop against which the understanding and cure of illness stand. The answer to the question "What is the matter?" dictates the reply to "What shall be done?" and both concerns must be viewed against what is generally believed about the nature of childhood.

Chapter 1, "Social Aspects," attempts to show the interplay of facts and beliefs in shaping certain social policies toward children. This chapter also emphasizes future directions and areas of special need, such as the importance of preventive intervention, the role of the classroom teacher in the recognition of symptoms, and the meanings of multiple-caretaking arrangements for the mental health of the young child.

Throughout the book, I attempt to give the student an overall picture of the nature of and approaches to child psychopathology, demonstrating through example the application of theory to technique and the importance of sound methods in diagnosis. Chapter 2, "Diagnostic Aspects," shows the spectrum of psychopathological disturbances. Then a detailed discussion of one type of psychosis is followed by a presentation of obsessive-compulsive neurosis through the case study of a young boy. Chapter 3, "Therapeutic Aspects," again presents a broad picture of the variety of approaches to child therapy, and then concentrates on the theories and techniques of four major approaches: psychoanalysis, intensive psychotherapy, family therapy, and educationally oriented residential treatment.

I wish to express my gratitude to my students and colleagues, as well as to those with whom I worked on the Joint Commission for the Mental Health of Children, for discussions and clarifications of the contents of this book. The completion of the manuscript was made easier by the painstaking and competent help of Mrs. Helen Rothberg, whose tactful suggestions were indispensable. I am also grateful to Jerome Kagan of Harvard University, Perry London of the University of Southern California, and

Joseph Lord of The Children's Hospital Medical Center (Boston) for their very helpful comments and suggestions on the manuscript.

Textbook writing is a form of teaching. Thus I owe a debt to all those who taught me well and made me a teacher. Their names appear on occasion in this book in the form of references or footnotes. Such conventions obscure the full meaning of seminars, discussions, and subsequent colleagueships with men and women who taught by taking all the risks of giving of themselves.

I have dedicated this book to the late Helen D. Sargent, whose supervision during my post-doctoral training at The Menninger Foundation influenced me profoundly. She communicated her values with passion and great intellectual clarity. Her conviction that working with children is the clinical psychologist's most challenging task; her belief that scientific facts must be viewed in their full ideological context, be that of the culture of science itself or of the larger society; her trust in the successful outcome of honest intellectual battles with recalcitrant complexities—all these made her a grand model for a clinical psychologist.

Mary Engel

Contents

CONTENTS

Prologue

This book begins with the case of a boy who was born to a widow. He came into the world in the fall of 1939, two months after the death of his father. He was the mother's third son. The first son was seven years older, of a previous marriage, and was thus half-brother to the boy. The second son was five years older and was the boy's full brother.

The mother had to go to work. She placed the two older boys in an orphans' home. The baby was cared for by the mother's older sister, by a neighbor, and some of the time by the mother herself. In 1942, when the boy was three years old, he too was sent to the orphanage. When he was five and a half the mother married, for the third time. She sent her two older sons to a military academy while the boy remained with her and his new stepfather. The boy got along well with his stepfather. In fact, he became attached to him. But when he was eight and a half the mother divorced the stepfather.

Following the divorce, the half-brother wanted to join the Marines. However, he was not yet seventeen years old. Nevertheless, the mother testified that he was of the required age. Then the mother went to work as a saleslady and often took the boy with her, leaving him in the car for long periods of time. Later, after he had started school, the boy would take care of himself in the mornings, at noon when he came home for lunch, and after school, and he learned to get his own meals. He did not play with other children. When he was eleven years old, he was sent to visit relatives in a distant city. The family noticed with some dismay that he was unwilling to play with children his own age.

By the time the boy was thirteen years old, the mother had decided to move to a large city to try her fortunes there. The boy and the mother moved east and took up residence with the eldest son, who was newly married. By this time there was evidence of the cumulative effect of the many changes in the boy's life. It is said that he struck his mother and threatened the young sister-in-law with a pocketknife during an argument. Soon the half-brother and his wife asked the mother and the boy to leave their home. Thereafter the boy refused to communicate with his half-brother, of whom he had previously been quite fond.

During this time, and in his fourteenth year, the boy was enrolled in the public school in the big city. Having come from the rural parts of the United States, he was subjected to much teasing from other children because of his strange accent and his rural clothes. He began to stay away from school and to remain at home, entertaining himself by reading magazines and watching television. Various probation officers tried at different times to convince him to return to school. Finally, truancy charges were brought against him and it was said that he was "beyond the control of his mother insofar as school attendance is concerned." He was sent for psychiatric observation to an institution in which children are often detained pending a court decision concerning them. He was there almost a month, during which time he was examined by the chief psychiatrist. The mother visited him there and later recalled the degradation of being searched "because the children in this home were such criminals, dope fiends, and had been in criminal offenses, that anybody entering this home had to be searched in case the parents were bringing in cigarettes or narcotics or anything." The boy pleaded with her, "Mother, I want to get out of here. There are children in here who have killed people, and smoke. I want to get out."

A somewhat different perspective on the boy comes from the recollections of his probation officer at the detention home, who thought the boy liked being there and did not miss his mother. The boy once told a social worker that the thing he disliked most about the detention home was that he always had to be with other children and that he dreaded their company, particularly when he had to undress in front of them.

The psychiatrist at the detention home recalled that the boy was tense, withdrawn, and evasive. He noticed the boy's preference for being alone, his evasion of the company of other children, and the difficulty he had in communicating. He said that the boy was withdrawn because of "intense anxiety, shyness, feelings of awkwardness and insecurity." The boy said to the psychiatrist, "I don't want a friend and I don't like to talk to people and I dislike everybody." The psychiatrist noted that the boy had an intense fantasy life and that in his fantasies he toyed with themes of omnipotence and power. The psychiatrist felt that these preoccupations were the boy's attempt to overcompensate for his basic feelings of inferiority. The summary of his report describes the boy as follows:

> This thirteen-year-old well-built boy has superior mental resources and functions only slightly below his

capacity level in spite of chronic truancy from school which brought him into Youth House. No findings of neurological impairment or psychotic mental changes could be made. [He] has to be diagnosed as "personality pattern disturbance with schizoid features and passive-aggressive tendencies." [The boy] has to be seen as an emotionally quite disturbed youngster who suffers under the impact of really existing emotional isolation and deprivation, lack of affection, absence of family life, and rejection by a self-involved and conflicted mother.

The psychiatrist suggested that the boy be placed on probation and treated in a child guidance clinic, that he be seen by a male psychiatrist, and that the mother be given psychotherapeutic guidance during this period of probation. It was decided not to commit the boy for institutional care until this plan was tried.

During the time of his evaluation the boy was additionally described by the social worker as a detached youngster who resented living by the rules of others and who avoided contact with people. However, she noted that there was about him "a rather pleasant, appealing quality," and she said that his emotional starvation and his affectionless life evoked from adults a kind of attraction and a wish to help him. She thought that the boy was quite convinced that his mother did not care about him, and that he always felt like a burden that had to be tolerated. At one time the boy told the social worker that he felt as if there were a veil between him and other people, that he wished to remain on one side of this veil, and that in his solitary position he often imagined that he was powerful enough to hurt and kill people. When asked to say more about these thoughts he withdrew into silence and declared them to be his own private business.

What was the mother like? We can assume that she had her share of difficulties. By the time the boy was thirteen and in serious trouble she had been twice divorced and once widowed, had had many jobs, and had changed her residence innumerable times, moving from one state to another as well as from one part of the country to another. Social workers associated with the boy have described her as a "smartly dressed, gray-haired woman, very self-possessed and alert and superficially affable . . . a rigid, self-involved person who had real difficulty in accepting and relating to people." The psychiatrist tried to explain to her that the boy's withdrawal was "a form of violent but silent protest against his neglect by her and [represented] his reactions to a complete absence of any real family life." Others who knew her thought that at certain times she spoiled the boy with excessive indulgence while at other times she rejected him. It is said that she slept in the same bed with the boy until he was close to eleven years old, a practice not often recommended by experts in child mental health. She was given to falsifying the birthdates of her children on public records when it suited her or their convenience and might thus have easily communicated to her sons that social institutions are to be betrayed.

At any event, one social worker's report about the boy at the age of thirteen sounded a serious note of warning as well as some hopeful tones:

> Despite his withdrawal, he gives the impression that he is not so difficult to reach as he appears, and patient, prolonged effort in a sustained relationship with one therapist might bring results. There are indications that he has suffered serious personality damage but if he can receive help quickly this might be repaired to some extent.

The serious personality damage was, however, never repaired. One child guidance agency did make an effort to help, but the mother never took advantage of the offer. Upon returning to school the boy again became a disciplinary problem, and the mother refused to cooperate with the school authorities. At this time placement in a home for boys was seriously considered, but before any court action was taken the mother took the boy out of the state; and in yet another school he finished the ninth grade. By his seventeenth birthday, when he joined the U.S. Marines, the boy had lived in twenty-three dwellings in five different cities, had been in an orphans' asylum and a detention home, and had attended twelve different schools while finishing nine grades.

He could hardly wait to join the Marines—he had tried to do so at the age of sixteen. He convinced his mother to falsify his age but failed to persuade the recruiter that he was seventeen, so his enlistment was postponed a year, during which time he attended no school but eagerly studied his brother's Marine Corps manual. It was his brother's opinion that the boy's eagerness to join the Marines had to do with his wish "to get from out and under the yoke of oppression" represented by the mother.

There is little use in documenting the remaining years of his young manhood, which appeared to be an extension of his earlier somberness, isolation, resentment of authority, and deeply lodged rage. The Marine Corps did not prove to be a solution for him. There he was seen as "a person who would go out of his way to get into trouble," and some thought he was subject to feelings of persecution, "a frail little puppy in the litter." Yet his tendency to challenge and provoke officers led to numerous clashes, one of which resulted in a court-martial hearing and a sentence of twenty-eight days.

At the age of twenty he left the Marine Corps and also left the United States. Those who knew him say that his defection to the Soviet Union was personal rather than ideological, but he was doomed to disappointment in Russia as well. When told that he could not remain there he attempted suicide; his diary at this time gives evidence of a near-psychotic state. And so it goes, through his marriage and eventual return to the United States. At the age of twenty-three, ten years after it had been said of him that he suffered serious personality damage still reparable by psychotherapy, after the orphanage, the detention home, and the twelve different schools, and after the Marines, the boy burned the full meaning of his psychopathology into the memory of a nation. On November 22, 1963, he assassinated President John F. Kennedy.[1]

Sometimes it takes a national tragedy to underline the full meaning of what is really already known. For many years professionals of all kinds have insisted that mental health services for children in the United States are dangerously inadequate. Social workers, pediatricians, clinical psychologists, educators, and administrators of health programs in various government agencies have long said that our country provides its youth with inferior, poorly coordinated services whose effect on the lives of children is not good enough and arrives too late. For years it has been said that the children who have the least get the least, that parents who experience the greatest difficulty raising their children and providing for them also have the least access to such services as do exist. People have always known that one kind of problem in growing up usually brings with it others. There has really been general agreement that when it comes to illness, physical or emotional, an ounce of prevention is worth a pound of cure. Clinicians have long been aware of the interrelationship between school failure, inferior home environment, and psychological problems in living. Various attempts have been made to take a look at the problems of children in the United States, but these attempts have been isolated and fragmented, reaching

[1] All facts and quotations pertaining to the life of Lee Harvey Oswald are taken from the *Report of the Warren Commission on the Assassination of President John F. Kennedy* (New York: Bantam Books, 1964).

limited audiences and seldom, it seems, catching the imagination of legislators.

The assassination of a beloved President and the subsequently discovered facts about the childhood of Lee Harvey Oswald mobilized considerable interest in the halls of government. People were beginning to raise anew questions that they had ceased asking; old anxieties about child welfare, child health, and above all child mental health reemerged. People wanted to know: How many such children may there be in our schools? What is being done for them? Does family break-up lead to mental illness in children? At what age "can you tell"? Are there effective cures and preventions? The list of questions was not a new one. But suddenly the death of the President and the life story of his assassin cast these old questions onto the large screen of national concern. Something had to be done.

While the nation was still in mourning, Senator Abraham Ribicoff of Connecticut introduced a bill in Congress providing for the creation of an organization composed of experts in child mental health and related fields, to be called the Joint Commission on Mental Health of Children.[2] The commission was charged with the task of studying all aspects of child mental illness in depth and delivering a set of recommendations to Congress. For over three years more than five hundred professionals from various disciplines—medicine, public health, psychology, social work, nursing, education, anthropology, and genetics—worked and wrote. All major aspects of child mental health were considered; all social institutions affecting the lives of children in the United States were scrutinized. People worked in teams as well as individually—some for several years, others for shorter periods of time—lending their expertise to the analysis of particu-

[2] Section 231(d) of the Social Security amendments of 1965 and 1968, P.L. 89–97.

lar kinds of problems. Thirteen national professional organizations cooperated, and the services of several educational and research organizations were enlisted and woven into the total effort.

The work of the Joint Commission on Mental Health of Children resulted in hundreds of pages of material consisting of descriptions of "how things are" as well as recommendations on "how things should be" in the lives of America's children. The first of several reports reached Congress in June 1969. In May 1970 the material started to become available to the general public through the first of a series of books. Under the title *Crisis in Child Mental Health* (1970), any citizen can now find the first and most thoroughly documented report substantiating the commission's main conclusion: the health and mental health care of children in the United States is in a deplorable condition, and nothing short of a major revision in services, education, research, and training of professionals will insure that the country's greatest natural resource, its child population, will get a sound start in life. All social institutions, such as prenatal clinics, hospitals, nursery schools, public schools, courts of law, detention homes, and adoption facilities, were found to be inadequate. In many cases they were seen as having a noxious effect on those they were supposed to help.

It is still too soon to tell what the effect of the work of the commission will be. This will depend on many factors, including national priorities, public sentiment, and the willingness of legislators to fight for the implementation of the recommendations that were made. Between the time of the commission's report to Congress and the writing of this book no major reconsideration of public policy toward children has been made. Some of us who worked hard and long on the Joint Commission on Mental Health of Children feel that the wind has gone out of our sails: How many years after we have done our reporting to Congress and to the nation will we see any changes in attitudes toward children?

And will these changed attitudes really result in sufficiently altered fiscal policies to permit implementation of some of our recommendations?

But as concerns shift and interests change, commitments may be realigned, and strong feelings may find new aims. With a deemphasis on the importance of material things may come new worries over the purity of the air, the beauty of the land, and the quality of life in the depths of the seas. Newly reordered priorities may make a place for renewed concern for the welfare of the nation's children. What happens to mentally ill children in the United States will depend also on the answer to a very simple question: Will the young people who read this book care deeply about those who are *even younger?*

CHAPTER ONE

Social
Aspects

Children in the news

An informed public is essential to the survival of a democracy. Many facts about mental illness in children reach the public not through textbooks but through the mass media. Magazines, television, radio, and newspapers have a powerful effect on public opinion. By the manner in which facts are presented and by the selection of facts for presentation, the media act as filtering lenses in the process of public information.

No adequate consideration of the social (societal) aspects of mental illness in children can be made without at least a brief look at the kinds of events related to the psychopathology of childhood that make news. During the past few years a reader of *The New York Times* might have seen several items relating to children, in particular a series of articles about child neglect and child abuse. For example, in the December 13, 1970, issue of *The New York Times* Robert Reinhold reported:

> . . . A major nationwide study has traced the high level of child-beating in this country to a widespread acceptance among Americans of the use of physical force as a legitimate procedure in child-rearing.
>
> This conclusion was reached by Dr. David G. Gil of Brandeis University after an analysis of 13,000 child-beating reports in all 50 states. It conflicts with past interpretations, which have generally attributed the abuse to the mental illness of the beater. . . . The "battered child syndrome," as the more severe forms of abuse are known, is one of the most perplexing problems facing health officials. Dr. Gil, who is a professor of social policy, estimated in an interview that as many as 2.5 million children are abused every year. However, reliable statistics are hard to obtain. . . . Bruises and welts were the most common type of injuries, followed by scratches and cuts. Other common injuries were burns and bone fractures.
>
> A majority of the 13,000 incidents reported in 1967 and 1968 were found to have resulted from "more or less acceptable disciplinary measures taken by caretakers in angry response to actual or perceived misconduct."

But lately the media have also reported cases of child abuse and neglect at the level of public institutions, suggesting that governmental bodies as well as private citizens are creating conditions that are deleterious to children. Consider the following quotation from an article by Robert E. Tomasson in the October 23, 1970, issue of *The New York Times:*

> . . . The Legal Aid Society filed suit here yesterday charging the city with widespread failure to provide

psychiatric care for hundreds of abandoned children in three city institutions.

In an unusual "class action," the society alleged that the "deleterious conduct [of the city] creates and perpetuates a vicious cycle in which abused and neglected children are deprived of badly needed treatment because they have the misfortune to reside in shelters which the city arbitrarily designates as 'temporary' residences." . . . At present, there are 468 children under the age of 16 being cared for in four city shelters. Yesterday's suit made no mention of Jennings Hall in Brooklyn, the newest of the city's shelters, which was opened last July. Two other institutions are in Manhattan and one is in Queens.

None of the four centers is overcrowded, according to the Department of Social Services.

Charles Schinitsky, who heads the Legal Aid Society's Family Court branch, alleged in the suit that while the centers had been designed for the temporary care of abandoned children until they could be placed in foster homes, they had become long-term custodial homes for children who were in desperate need of psychiatric care, which they were not receiving.

In his petition to the court, Mr. Schinitsky briefly outlined the background of eight children of whom he had been appointed the legal guardian after they had been abandoned by their parents.

Three of the four children mentioned in the suit are Robert, seven years old, who was "unable to utter an intelligible sentence"; Michael, eight, a schizophrenic who received no special treatment; and 15-year-old Bonita, who was described as having "neurotic depression with borderline features."

Such news items probably affect most citizens deeply. Letters-to-the-editor sections in newspapers testify to the occasional outrage felt by teacher and parent groups. There is ample evidence that adults do band together and do get things done for children, and that such group action takes place with increasing frequency, although the methods necessary to bring about change are often rather extreme. Juan M. Vasquez wrote in the November 6, 1970, issue of *The New York Times:*

> The city promised yesterday to finance fully or in part nine day-care centers operating under the principle of community control.
>
> Jule M. Sugarman, who heads the Human Resources Administration, told representatives of the nine centers that money would be made available by next Friday.
>
> His meeting with the group followed a three-hour occupation of H.R.A. headquarters by 100 mothers, teachers, and children demanding funds to operate the centers.

From sit-ins and fights over day care facilities to complaints about child abuse and public criticism about educational and welfare programs, it is not far to concerted and serious political action. Programs require money. There is not enough money. There are loud disagreements over how the money should be spent. Serious questions are raised about national priorities. These questions are often posed in polarized terms. For example, a recent and angry exchange in the letters-to-the-editor section of *Life* magazine concerned the question: Should the country spend more of its resources on the care of old people, or should more money be spent on the welfare of children and youth? The argument arose over an article about day care facilities (*Life,* July 31, 1970) written by Mrs. Richard Lansburgh, president of the Day Care and Child Development Council of America. She wrote that the United States spends nine dollars on every aging person for every dollar spent on a child. She questioned the wisdom of this disproportionality because of the generally poor services offered to children. Then John B. Martin, special assistant to the President on the problems of aging, offered several counterarguments. He pointed out that children and young people have their parents to depend on, whereas old people, who suffer from many kinds of illness, frequently have no one to turn to. Reply was then made by Mrs. Lansburgh, showing that a disproportionate number of children under six years of age live in poverty and that it is therefore not fair to assume that simply because they are children they have economic and social supports. She pointed out that according to the 1969 report of the Bureau of the Census 48 percent of the *poor* in metropolitan areas were under the age of eighteen and 18 percent were under the age of six.

One cannot long discuss the problems of child health and mental health without finding oneself fully involved in the largest social questions of the day. Many discussions begin with child mental health and end in disagreements over appropriations for highways, aircraft, and war. Meetings with ostensibly scientific purposes often become political rallies, and professors as well as clinical psychologists are quickly drawn into participation in social pressure groups such as the children's lobby in New York City.[1]

It is difficult to construct a sound and considered position with regard to problems of child health and mental health purely on the basis of facts offered by the public media. News items give quick information. Even when the information is accurate (which often is not the case), its context is necessarily limited. Moreover, serious problems of interpretation arise over even the most accurate facts. All decisions based on facts have moral as well as political implications.

[1] See *The New York Times*, Sunday, December 13, 1970, p. 1.

The assumption behind this book is that it is important for students of human behavior not only to understand problems pertaining to the gathering of facts but also to be acquainted with the complexities of social action taken on the basis of facts. These complexities consist of historical and economic realities often not well known by the general public. Yet without such understanding, rational discourse and serious explanation soon deteriorate into empty shouting. It is the children who suffer. For example, a recent report from the U.S. Department of Health, Education, and Welfare states:

> An estimated 500,000 American children are afflicted with psychoses and borderline psychotic conditions. Another million suffer from other severe mental disorders. Of the 50 million elementary school children in the United States, it is estimated that between 10 and 12 percent have moderate to severe emotional problems requiring some kind of mental health care. Among the 15 million youngsters in the United States who are being reared in poverty, one out of three has emotional problems that need attention. The number of young patients being admitted to mental hospitals is increasing steadily. Many long-term patients were first admitted as children or young adults. Drug abuse and delinquency are growing problems. Less than one percent of the disturbed youngsters in the United States receive any kind of treatment, and less than half of these receive adequate help.[2]

These are facts. The mere awareness of them will make little difference in the lives of children. Facts have to be translated into

[2] National Clearing House for Mental Health Information, *The National Institute of Mental Health*, Information Publication No. 5027 (Washington, D.C.: U.S. Government Printing Office, 1970), p. 7.

social action. And social action is determined by public policy, which both rests on and creates public opinion.

Public policy and the problem of facts

Public policy is a collection of decisions and practices. In the area of child mental health, these decisions determine what kinds of services should be available to children and how much money will be spent on such services. Public policy decisions also determine in what manner the services should be made available, through what channels, and under what regulations. In a democracy it is very difficult to ascertain how public policy is made. In countries that have an administrative structure known as the Ministry of Child Health, we would say that the minister makes the final decisions, and we could probably name a few other people around him who advise him. In our country the process (and power) of decision-making is much more widely spread. As one government official recently put it:

> The formation of public policy is a highly complex process. For most child development programs it involves a whole series of judgments and decisions within one or more Cabinet departments, followed by reconsideration and redecision at the Budget Bureau and perhaps in the White House. Finally, there is congressional reconsideration and redecision, which usually involve action by at least four committees, both houses in the Congress, a conference committee, and, once again, both houses. At each stage, there are intelligent and informed officials who are well acquainted with the reports of the media and who base much of their

thinking on the media reports, from which they may
also get much of their information. . . .[3]

It is clear from this brief description of the process by which
public policy is made that facts are not the sole determinants of
what laws are written, how much tax money is appropriated, and
what national priorities are chosen. The media, public opinion,
and public belief are also powerful factors in influencing public
policy. Nevertheless, facts and the accuracy of facts do make a
difference. The compilation of data is often the business of re-
searchers, or of professionals invited to advise the government
about existing conditions. So it was with the Joint Commission on
Mental Health of Children, formed in 1968. Many of the facts
related to child mental health quoted in this book were gathered
by that commission. What this writer knows about the problem
of gathering socially relevant facts was learned during her years
of service on the commission.

One of the most interesting considerations in the formulation
of public policy in the field of mental health is that it inevitably
involves the cooperation of scientists and politicians. Scientists
are concerned with what is known, how more can be known,
and what the areas of uncertainty of knowledge are. Those in
government represent the "doing" side of the enterprise. They
know how to write a bill, when to present it, and how to persuade others to support it; they know how much money can be
asked for and can anticipate the arguments of opponents. Thus
both scientists and legislators are essential if tax dollars are to be
spent on behalf of mentally ill children.

It is necessary that scientists understand the problems of
legislators and that lawmakers have at least a good layman's
understanding of the issues that scientists raise. The problems

[3] Jule M. Sugarman, "Research, evaluation, and public policy,"
Child Development, 41 (1970), 263–66.

that arise in this area have been expertly considered by the British physicist, writer, and statesman C. P. Snow (1960). Snow focused on the "two-culture problem" in Britain and cited as a primary example the struggle between Sir Henry Tizard, a leader in the development of radar, and F. A. Lindemann, Winston Churchill's scientific adviser. In this instance the conflict between the scientist and the politician could easily have cost Britain its survival.

Fearing that England was vulnerable to air attack, the British Air Ministry created a scientific advisory committee to investigate the possibilities of using scientific and technical knowledge to defend the country against hostile aircraft. Sir Henry Tizard was among the distinguished scientists who served on the committee, which began to deliberate in 1935. Churchill, who maintained that the government underestimated the size of Hitler's air force, insisted that F. A. Lindemann sit with the Tizard committee. Lindemann was a physicist, but scientists had little respect for his accomplishments and regarded him as a politician, and in those years a not very important politician at that.

The members of the Tizard committee resented the presence of Lindemann in their midst. He in turn resented the influence and prestige of the committee. Tizard and the others held to the view that radar defense was England's only hope. Lindemann had a pet device of his own, infra-red detection. He also believed in dropping parachute bombs on hostile aircraft. The committee saw these suggestions as impractical, as indeed in the long run they turned out to be.

The Tizard-Lindemann feud continued for one year. Several members resigned from the committee, despairing of ever reaching an agreement. It was not until the committee was reappointed and Lindemann was replaced by E. V. Appleton, a physicist who had done extensive work on radio waves, that the matter of the air defense of England was finally decided in favor of radar.

As this example illustrates, the difficulties of formulating public policy are not confined to education or mental health. Rather these difficulties have features that transcend what a specific kind of public policy is *about* and reside in the divergent ways of thinking on the part of scientists and politicians.

For example, while scientists are trained to doubt and to present their results with due qualification, legislators cannot survive with such an attitude toward facts. Scientists are trained to test their results many times before they believe that "it is so." Legislators have to catch the swing of the moment and to implement—to make happen—what they advocate. Often the doubts of scientists seem strange, obsessive, and excessive to lawmakers, while scientists sometimes shudder at the speed and conviction with which scientific facts enter the mainstream of public life. Although this is perhaps an oversimplification, not allowing for individual differences among scientists and lawmakers, it should serve to point up the fact that there is an *essential stress* in the process of formulating public policy about mentally ill children that is not peculiar to this area.

The child labor laws enacted in the United States toward the end of the last century are a clear example of our public policy toward children. In 1870 the federal census reported that the number of working children between the ages of ten and fifteen had reached about 750,000. By the turn of the century the number had risen to 1,750,000. The Children's Aid Society refuted these figures, pointing out that in New York City alone there were at least 100,000 children between the ages of eight and sixteen who were working.

In the mines and in the streets, in garment factories and in brickyards, as beggars, musicians, and bootblacks, children worked under conditions that we now consider criminal and cruel. But during most of the nineteenth century there was no public policy, no law, no regulation. Factory owners could hire children and abuse them with impunity; parents could force their children to work in subhuman conditions. Whatever children thought about all this remains a mystery for the most part. Children cannot vote, have no money, and cannot travel. For such reasons they have no political power and very little power over their own lives.

Child labor laws as we know them today were enacted in response to public outrage about the lives of children who grew up under these conditions. In some ways the laws were very effective. In other ways they failed to address themselves to the basic causes of the abuse of child workers. In still other ways they are unenforceable and in a sense overshoot the mark. It can be shown, for example, that there are features of early work experience that are not *in themselves* harmful to children.[4]

The United States, of course, has not been alone in generating public policies about youngsters. The Binet Intelligence Test for children was developed in 1904 by Alfred Binet, who was commissioned by the French government to devise ways by which intellectually slow pupils could be identified in the schools. The techniques became a well-known intelligence test, and the IQ score was applied to thousands of children in both Europe and America, though not at all in the manner in which Alfred Binet intended. In 1911 Binet complained bitterly about the uses to which his "tests" were being put and cautioned educators not to regard any child's score as an inherent or unalterable sign of intellectual limitation. He pointed out that schoolmasters were using the IQ score as a punitive label, neglecting the fact that there are many reasons why children fail to learn in school. Binet called on educators to realize that the intelligence test performance of any child reflected, at least in part, how well he had been taught—that is, Binet viewed *intelligence test scores as mirroring*

---

[4] The study of the psychological aspects of early work experience has recently begun. See, for example, M. Engel, "Children who work," *Archives of General Psychiatry,* 17 (1967), 291–97.

the quality of the schools. He began to call attention to the fact that some children were not able to learn because they had devastating experiences with their teachers and pointed out that poverty, malnutrition, and deprivation were also factors accounting for low intelligence. Binet urged teachers to keep in mind that some children *could not learn,* whereas others *would not be taught.* But for the most part his warnings fell on deaf ears, and the IQ score soon became a much abused and misunderstood psychological datum about children.[5]

The enactment of child labor laws in the United States was the result of a long process of public policymaking. It received momentum from facts about the kinds of abuse inflicted upon children of different ages by various employers. By contrast, Binet's mission was to generate facts on the basis of which public policy decisions could be made. Such facts as the conditions under which children are made to work, or their physical and intellectual abilities, differ with regard to precision in that personal judgments are always less involved when known procedures of measurement are used. But values are heavily involved whenever facts are gathered. Values dictate what facts are worth knowing. The kinds of facts we collect contain a prophecy: someone, somehow, wants to do something that might affect large segments of the population.

Public policies affect children's lives by prohibiting or altering existing practices or by initiating new procedures. Child labor laws are an example of prohibition, or at least of severe restriction. The development of the Binet scales in France represents an alteration of existing practices. The creation of day care centers in the United States today is an example of initiating new procedures. In all three cases, the relationship between facts and the policies based on them is fairly complex; facts are tied to

[5] See A. Binet, *Les idées modernes sur les enfants* (Paris: Flammarion, 1911).

action by values, commitments, anxieties, beliefs, and assumptions. Few of these are usually verbalized. In heated discussions about the relative wisdom of some public action over another, problems pertaining to facts are themselves often confused with questions of value.

There are essentially two major problems about facts: their accuracy and their relevance. The accuracy of some facts is durable, whereas a large number of facts are only temporarily accurate. In complex social realities many things are true today but not tomorrow. Some matters may be accurately assessed, but the assessment hinges so much on context, that when the context changes the facts are no longer as true as they were before, or indeed they may have become fiction. Facts gathered in the service of remedying complex social problems are often outdated before action based upon them can take place.

Suppose you were to interview members of a housing project in a part of town inhabited by a racial or ethnic minority. Your purpose is to reach an intelligent decision on the question: Can a social worker from the dominant cultural group be employed in this community and would such a person be accepted? You are earnest. You do not want to act without facts. Your study is carefully done and your subjects well selected, and you conclude from your data that the plan would indeed work—the community is receptive to the idea and needs the help you are going to offer.

But as you prepare to act on your conclusion, a serious event takes place in the community. Local groups feel themselves insulted by a member of the majority culture. The community turns bitter, resentful. It does not want help from you or from any outsider. It seems best not to do anything for the moment. Your facts were accurate but only as long as the context remained unaltered. This example is an extreme one, to be sure, but it serves to underline the chameleon-like quality of facts in social science and the delicate relationship between their accuracy and their context.

Some facts are accurate relative to a certain part of the country, to a particular segment of the population, or to a fixed span of time. While most social scientists agree on this, they find it very difficult not to reify facts, not to give them an absolute "hard and fast" quality. In truth, one cannot always keep the transitory accuracy of facts fully in mind. If the world is always in quotation marks, how can one reach decisions, or even believe in the possibility of solving complex social problems? Thus we often act as though facts were more lastingly accurate than we know them to be, and we allow ourselves this luxury in order to be able to act at all.

Another problem with facts is their relevance. In the example above, you would also have to decide *what you needed to know that would help you determine* the kind of person the community would accept. You could gather many accurate facts—the ages of the residents, the sizes of the families, and so on—that would not be likely to change with shifts of emotions. But would these facts help you in deciding on some social action? Might there not be some other, more relevant facts? For example, perhaps it would help to know who the leader in the community was and what his beliefs were. Decisions about the relevance of facts are often based on previous experience, on hypotheses, or on insights. The less previous knowledge there is, the greater the role that personal values play in taking sides and choosing positions about social action.

If teachers always kept all these qualifications in mind, teaching facts would be even more difficult than it is.[6] Textbook writing would be even more impossible. With all this in mind, let us now consider some facts pertaining to child mental illness that in this writer's judgment are reasonably accurate and relevant at this time. The reader will no doubt find much ground for argu-

---

[6] Sigmund Freud once wrote that there are three impossible professions: teaching, curing, and governing.

ment and disagreement over public policies in the making. It is hoped that some of the facts presented here will be helpful in guiding thought and judgment about the mental health issues of today and tomorrow.[7]

An ounce of prevention

According to the report of the Bureau of the Census, the population of the United States in 1970 was 203,184,772.[8] Of this population, 93,350,853 people were under twenty-five years of age. That is, young people comprised 45.92 percent of the population. When these young people are grouped according to certain characteristics, some interesting facts begin to emerge. In 1970, 87 percent of the youth in America were white and 64 percent lived in or close to urban centers. The age distribution within the youth population was fairly even, as shown below:

AGE	PERCENTAGE OF POPULATION
20–25	8.05
15–19	9.38
10–14	10.23
5–9	9.82
under 5	8.44

[7] Additional facts on mental illness in children may be found in the Joint Commission on Mental Health of Children, *Crisis in Child Mental Health* (New York: Harper and Row, 1970), as well as in the various government publications referred to throughout this book.

[8] Population statistics are taken from *Current Population Reports,* Series P-20, No. 197 (March 1970), Census Library, Federal Plaza, New York, N.Y.

Even if we had no other information except these figures, we might begin to reason that public policymakers should spend at least as much money on young people as on those who are older than twenty-five. It would also appear that urban youth should be in the forefront of political considerations. But as we shall see below, age and residence are not the only important factors.

There is in public health the concept of the *high-risk group.* This term means that some people are more likely than others to become ill. The identification of high-risk groups is a matter of great concern; many arguments about the choice of a right course of action really originate in *differing procedures in the methods of defining high-risk groups.*

One common way of defining high-risk groups, from the point of view of mental health, is by age. That is, one can think through the age span of childhood and ask: At what times in their lives are children exposed to greater mental health risks than at other times? Another way to define high-risk groups is by circumstance. Here one asks: Is it possible to identify segments of the population whose members are exposed to high health risks, regardless of their age or developmental status? Most frequently, these two approaches intertwine, as will be seen in the example below.

It has been shown that babies born out of wedlock constitute a high-risk group, from the point of view of mental health. Their number has risen from below 90,000 in 1940 to over 290,000 in 1965. Their mothers constitute a large proportion of those women who attempt to raise their children without the aid and protection of a husband. Two-thirds of all unwed mothers are living below the poverty line. These women are a very diverse group—there is no such thing as a "personality type" among unwed mothers. But numerous factors converge to render these babies and their mothers worthy of special attention in planning mental health services.

Women who are expecting a baby out of wedlock are less likely to receive good medical care during pregnancy. There are several reasons for this. Many unwed mothers are teenagers who shy away from medical clinics that are not geared to understanding their problems. Even in these days of sexual emancipation, a good deal of shame is attached to the mother's situation. Social institutions do not exactly seek out unwed mothers for special care; rather the tone toward them tends to be punitive and moralistic. Consider these facts in light of some others concerning the importance of the mother's physical and emotional condition during pregnancy.

The most important time, from the point of view of the baby's brain development, is the first trimester of pregnancy. Bleeding, toxemia, infection, and malnutrition are some of the dangers to the developing fetus during this time. To the extent that unwed mothers are less likely to receive adequate medical care during pregnancy, their babies' chances for good mental and physical health are already inferior to those of other babies. There are, of course, innumerable examples of the interplay between poor health and poor mental health. It is now known that there is an infernal intercorrelation between poverty, urban living, nonwhite racial background, and all kinds of indices of "high risk."

On the whole, compared with other nations the United States ranks very low in the quality of care it extends to mothers and babies around the time of birth. A crude and grim index of this inadequate care is the fact that the United States ranks thirteenth in infant mortality, with a rate of 24.7 deaths per thousand live births. This is twice the rate of Sweden and one-and-a-half times that of Japan!

Not only do other countries outstrip the United States in terms of low infant mortality; they also take better care of the mothers and babies who do survive. It has long been known that prematurely born babies constitute a high-risk group, requiring special preventive intervention. Of course, the best form of intervention is to reduce the number of premature live births. That is, the earlier help is given, the more effective it is, from both the general health and the mental health point of view. Prematurity often brings with it minimal forms of physical damage and physical incapacity. From the mental health point of view, these may become critical determinants of poor self-esteem. For example, minimal brain damage need not be totally incapacitating, but it may, in interaction with other factors such as poor schools and poor teaching, lead to problems in reading or arithmetic. These in turn may lead to a sense of failure, anxiety, and adjustment problems of various sorts. Those who believe in preventive intervention point out how much better it would be to reduce the number of premature births rather than to try to provide remedial and psychotherapeutic help for children with learning problems after their difficulties in school have manifested themselves.

It goes without saying that prematurity does not necessarily lead to adjustment problems. There are degrees of prematurity. Seven out of every hundred babies are born prematurely (that is, under five-and-a-half pounds), but some are smaller, or more premature, than others. In addition, the risks of prematurity are correlated with factors associated with poverty and social deprivation. When care is poor and life circumstances are harsh, prematurity becomes a greater single risk to mental health than any other antecedent to mental illness.

For a long time there were no precise ways to quantify the condition of babies as they arrived into the world. Today hospitals have begun to rate the newborn on five characteristics, according to a system developed by the pediatrician Virginia Apgar. These characteristics, known in abbreviated form as APGAR ratings, are as follows: appearance, pulse, grimace, activity, and respiration. Each attribute is rated on a one-to-ten-point scale by the nurse immediately after birth. The system has the dual advantage of shifting more attention from the mother to the baby in the delivery room and of recording for the baby's future some very relevant facts about his condition at the time of birth. By the end of this decade each youngster should have on his hospital record a numerical expression of his state of health at birth.

The power of circumstance

The above discussion is intended to show that the circumstances of children and their families have a powerful effect upon their mental health and/or that the status of their mental and physical health is also an expression of the quality of the early environment. While most people recognize the cyclical nature of the problem of poverty and mental health, they tend to think that poverty is more of a determinant of mental health than mental health is a determinant of economic status.

The term *poverty* is a very general one. In 1968 the U.S. Department of Labor estimated that an urban worker with a wife and two children would need an annual income of $9,150 a year to maintain a "modest but adequate" living standard. This figure is very relative, however, not only to the status of inflation but also to the geographical location of the family. Even among communities classified as "urban" there is a wide range in living costs. In 1969 the Joint Commission on Mental Health of Children recommended the guidelines for defining poverty that appear in the table on page 30.[9]

These income figures are certainly not worth memorizing. They will soon be out of date. But they illustrate the importance of *gradations of poverty* and suggest that arguments in which "the poor" are discussed as a homogeneous group are likely not to make any sense at all.

[9] Income figures are from *Current Population Reports, Consumer Income*, Series P-60, No. 72 (August 1970), Census Library, Federal Plaza, New York, N.Y.

INCOME CATEGORY	INCOME RANGE IN DOLLARS	PERCENTAGE OF POPULATION IN 1969 (BY HOUSEHOLDS)
Critically poor	less than 2,000	10.0
Seriously poor	2,000–4,000	12.4
Marginally poor	4,000–6,000	11.7
Inadequate income	6,000–8,000	13.2
Adequate income	8,000–10,000	12.9
Highly adequate income	10,000–12,000 ⎫	
Comfortable	12,000–15,000 ⎭	23.1
Prosperous	15,000 and over	16.6

While it is correct to say that in 1969 households in or below the inadequate-income category comprised 47.3 percent of all households in this country, the heterogeneity of the people—from the psychological as well as the economic point of view—must be taken into account. With regard to family style, level of aspiration, and child-raising beliefs—factors associated with racial and ethnic background—the poor are a very diverse group. Economic realities in interaction with these many personal factors create a multivariate picture the complexity of which we are just now beginning to understand. The more one knows about the interrelated factors of poverty the more cautious one becomes in presenting recommendations for lawmakers.

Let us look at some of the correlates of poverty that lead to the inference that poor health and poor mental health are the closest neighbors of the poor. Following are selected quotes from the report of the Joint Commission on Mental Health of Children:

> Although a number of factors other than psychological
> ones play into the incidence of school failure, early
> school dropout, unemployment, juvenile delinquency,

drug addiction, family breakdown, and illegitimacy, the far higher rates of these problems for poor people indicate, among other things, the corrosive impact of poverty on the mental health of children and youth in low income families. (p. 184.)

Of the estimated 3 per cent of children and youth who are mentally retarded, 75 per cent show no obvious brain damage and have few physical handicaps. Typically, these nonorganic cases come from census tracts where the median income is $3,000 per year or less. (p. 184.)

There is a consistent correlation between poverty and the number of school dropouts. Of the million youths who will drop out of school this year, about 65 per cent will come from families with incomes of less than $5,000; about 85 per cent from families with incomes of less than $7,500. (p. 185.)

The most important single factor associated with family breakdown is poverty itself. (p. 197.)

Most of the 600,000 children between the ages of three and five who attended Head Start programs in 1965 had never been to a physician or dentist and had not received immunization. . . . Black children receive about half as much attention from doctors as white children. (p. 201.)

Problems of unemployment are particularly critical for youths between the ages of sixteen and nineteen. In 1967 the unemployment rate for blacks in this age group was almost 30 per cent compared to 10 per cent for whites. . . . The employment problems of poor people, especially of the nonwhite poor, have a severe impact on the well-being of children and youth. (pp. 202–03.)

Professionals in the health sciences often complain that between the time of birth and entrance into school or kindergarten children disappear from public view. That is, after infants are taken home from the hospital there is no single social institution that consistently monitors their fate—unless of course a child commits a crime and his parents are brought to court. But in most cases children are left entirely to the mercy of whatever good or bad fortune befalls them. It is often said that since development is very vulnerable during the preschool years, society should insure that babies and toddlers remain in public view. Some kind of records should be kept on all children, and those who are exposed to malnutrition, poor care, or health and mental health risks of all sorts should be tagged as members of a high-risk group. Society should then intervene in their lives, on their best behalf. It is easy to see the reasoning behind this argument. Nothing can be prevented if it is not known, no noxious circumstance can be improved if its existence is entirely private, no child can be protected if he is anonymous. Yet there are equally strong arguments against such societal monitoring. As one expert in mental health said:

> . . . The "monitoring" or listing of children at the local level . . . has been soft-pedaled because of concern about the invasion of privacy and other problems which good-hearted computers might get into. I am not impressed with the compassion of computers, nor with their concern for individual liberties.[10]

[10] Comments by Dr. Dane Prugh, former president of the American Orthopsychiatric Association, in *Frontiers of Hospital Psychiatry*, 7 (1970), 2.

It should be noted that those who debate the wisdom and desirability of "tagging" children during the early preschool years have in mind more than just protecting children from obvious neglect, abuse, and cruelty. Their major concern is with identifying children whose chances are poor *before* they become either mentally or physically ill. At this time no such method for early identification has been found, except perhaps greater emphasis on mental health principles in the training of pediatricians who work in well-baby clinics. But one has reason to be skeptical; well-baby clinics are very busy places and often there is just minimal time to talk to the mother about her child. Is it really possible to make a sound judgment about the total health status of the family in such a setting?

How many are not like the others?

By the time children enter public school, many of their mental health problems are consolidated and begin to find expression in overt behavior—in the inability to learn, concentrate, or form good relationships with teachers and other children. Studies of maladjustment in school-age children show certain regularities; that is, we can generalize from their findings and reach some conclusions regarding the mental health status of America's schoolchildren. Note, however, that in order to accept any of these generalizations we must settle for a very broad meaning of the term *maladjustment* and regard it not as a diagnostic category but as a loose label covering lagging behind one's age mates, lacking in self-discipline, and behaving strangely.

Once children have entered school, the primary person who judges them is the teacher. Teachers not only rate academic performance. As a group they are in an excellent position to notice health and mental health problems in children. After all, they know hundreds of youngsters of the same age, and regardless of the quality of their training they do develop a frame of reference about what is expectable behavior and what is deviant, aberrant, or peculiar. It is a well-known fact that in clinical work teachers are the most frequent sources of referral. Typically, teachers become concerned about certain children and talk to the parents or to the guidance counselor; some of the children are then brought to clinics or mental health centers for further study. How sound or valid are these initial judgments of teachers? A host of studies show that teachers and clinical child psychologists and psychiatrists agree on 70 to 80 percent of their judgments about maladjustment in children. This degree of agreement is as good as any we might expect among clinicians.[11]

The relationship between parents' views of maladjustment of their children and teachers' judgments is high and statistically significant *if* the social class of the children is taken into account. The correlation is quite high (.90 in one study) between parents and teachers of middle class children. With lower class children the correlation drops (.17 in one study). It might be proposed that the reason for this discrepancy is that teachers have a tendency to overemphasize the pathological meaning of aggressive behavior, which is assumed to be more prevalent among poor children. But this does not appear to be the case. However, teachers are much more concerned about withdrawn behavior in girls than are lower class mothers, and this accounts for much of the discrepancy in judgment.

In general, there does seem to be a relationship between low intellectual performance and teachers' judgment of maladjustment, but the same is not true in reverse. In several studies poor

[11] All facts pertaining to the identification of maladjustment in schoolchildren are from J. C. Glidewell, "The prevalence of maladjustment in elementary schools," a report prepared in December 1967 for the Joint Commission on Mental Health of Children.

school achievement in the elementary grades was related to judgments of poor adjustment made by teachers when the children were older, but the children so rated did not have lower intelligence than classmates who were rated as well adjusted.

It is clear from a number of studies that women teachers perceive a greater degree of maladjustment in boys than in girls. However, when most of these studies were done, there were so few male teachers that it was impossible to make meaningful comparisons between male and female teachers on their view of maladjustment.

In general, teachers rate more lower class than middle class children as maladjusted. This fact is very difficult to interpret. Most teachers have grown up in middle class homes, and those who have not usually adhere strongly to middle class values. Moreover, until recently hospitals, clinics, and child guidance centers "favored" middle class patients. Thus it is misleading to simply count the number of child patients from different social classes in measuring the distribution of mental illness. For example, in 1964 the U.S. Population Reference Bureau found that almost twice as many middle class white children were receiving psychotherapy as lower class white children or black children. But the data used in this study were gathered from clinical facilities that were costly to patients and that often required that the child come from an intact family and that the father as well as the mother be involved in counseling or therapy. (Rosen, Bahn, and Kramer, 1964.)

In spite of these difficulties in obtaining good facts, can we estimate the degree of maladjustment in the school population of the United States? Glidewell (1967) has summarized twenty-nine studies of maladjustment in children done between 1922 and 1966. These studies concerned pupils from kindergarten through the eighth grade who resided mainly in the East and the Midwest. All the studies relied on teacher judgments to a large degree. From them Glidewell was able to generalize that about 30 percent of all children in elementary school were seen as presenting some psychological problem or another, and of these 9 percent presented problems serious enough for clinical intervention. Of the latter group 2 to 3 percent were actually referred to a clinic or hospital; the rest went untreated. About 1 percent of all boys were judged to be psychotic. Only .3 percent of all girls were found to be suffering from some kind of psychotic disorder. But this estimate of prevalence has to be taken with a grain of salt. As mentioned before, the cost of psychiatric care and the admission requirements of some clinics do not allow an accurate estimate.

At any event, in 1960 there were 30 million schoolchildren between five and twelve years of age. Of these 2.7 million needed the help of a psychologist or psychiatrist. Three times as many boys as girls in each grade presented mental health problems. An overall estimate was as follows: 14 percent of all boys and 5 percent of all girls were in need of some professional attention; 6 percent of all boys and 2 percent of all girls would have been sent to a clinic or hospital if such facilities had been available to the extent to which they were needed.

Glidewell concludes tentatively that when social class differences among children are held constant, racial differences in maladjustment are nil. That is, on dimensions such as "acceptance of authority" and "ability to concentrate" lower class children fare worse than middle class youngsters, and this is true for black as well as white children. Middle class black children act more like middle class white children than like lower class black children.

To sum up a complex network of findings, Glidewell concludes that 9 *percent is the best estimate for the prevalence of maladjustment in the middle years of childhood.* This is very close to the range of 10 to 12 percent prevalence given by the National Institute of Mental Health for moderate to severe emotional problems in school-age children.

Predictions for the future are fairly grim. Consider one example. It is estimated that by 1980 children and youth will represent half the population of the United States. Since at present more than 500,000 children are brought to court each year for antisocial acts, and an equal number suffer from psychoses, the continued expansion of the youth population forecasts a decrease in the quality of service to children. Since hospitals, courts, rehabilitation services, psychiatric clinics, and medical care facilities are already scarce; since the rate of training of professionals falls far short of the need; and since all institutions serving children are already of marginal quality and inadequate capacity, it is difficult to rejoice in the thought that children and youth might be increasing in number. Yet they are the country's greatest and most valuable resource.

These facts and predictions create deep apprehension among those who work with children in the mental health fields. Some redouble their efforts in basic research, with the conviction that too little is known to act wisely on behalf of large groups of children. They believe that the present state of knowledge in psychology, psychiatry, and medicine is far from ready for practical implementation. From this vantage point it would appear that the researcher-turned-social-activist contributes to the destruction of the generation of knowledge. If he could control his "do-goodism" and stay in his laboratory, he would be more useful and might discover new techniques of prevention, new methods of education, better drugs, and new cures.

Others in the field of mental health believe that the only way to really find out how to help people is to start helping them. They feel that findings from the laboratory might be useful in controlling physical diseases, but that mental illness is the result of a complex of social factors that can never be studied in the laboratory. Thus knowledge applicable to human relationships has to be generated by relating to people with problems. Still others feel that the root of all these problems is in misplaced national priorities. They seek remedies in the political arena. They point out that when $400 is spent for each citizen's defense and $13 for each citizen's health, no amount of knowledge can ever be implemented. Finally, there are those who believe that knowledge and funds together will not help if there are not enough trained professionals to deliver services to children and families. These people place their faith in youth and continue to teach.

Public policy and public belief:
the changing image of the child

The decisions that adults make about children are never based only on facts and are indeed often difficult to understand unless they are placed in the context of different cultural values and beliefs about the nature of childhood. As we will see below, the concept of the child as a person whose mental health may be in danger is a relatively recent one and is still not generally accepted. The following section traces the evolution of the idea of childhood in Western Europe and America and considers the idea of childhood in contemporary societies whose public policies toward children are markedly different from our own.

Social scientists have not yet achieved a precise understanding of the manner in which various concepts of the nature of the child gain expression in public policy. Yet, as we shall see, public convictions, ideas, beliefs, and values about children do play an important part in determining what public action is taken. For example, when a child's aberrant behavior is seen as a sign of his evil nature—because the society regards children as unsocialized monsters—punitive action is likely to result. When aberrant behavior is seen as a symptom of psychological disturbance—because the society believes that children are emotionally vulnerable and psychologically sensitive—remedial or therapeutic efforts are likely to result. But what if there is no public consensus, but rather indecision and ambivalence? Cultures as well as individuals are remarkably adept at finding compromise solutions that cater to several different values, beliefs, and convictions at once. If we cannot decide whether a child's behavior is "crazy" or "bad," we may prescribe policies that are an expression of both—our wish to cure and our need to punish. Or, if there is sufficient ambivalence about these matters, we may do nothing.

It is the thesis of this discussion that for very good reasons residing in history contemporary attitudes about mental illness in children are fraught with contradictions. Children symbolize many aspects of the human condition about which we are divided: the acceptability of free impulse expression and the advantages of self-control; the relative value of dependence and independence from parents; the importance of play over the importance of work; the comparative virtues of uniqueness and of conformity. Little wonder that children whose behavior is especially anxiety-ridden, strange, erratic, and annoying to adults elicit destructive as well as benign reactions from society.

The value and meaning of the child—a look into the past

If you asked a random sample of adults today what they believe and value about children, you would probably conclude that this is the "century of the child," that youngsters are treasured and respected and are regarded as very important and central in the life of the family. If you took care to interview special segments of the population, like suburban housewives or upper middle class parents, you could increase the likelihood of obtaining rather solid agreement that the careful raising of children is a mission and a duty, pleasurable and "fun."

The centrality of the child in the family is, however, a relatively recent development. In the Middle Ages childhood was very short, compared with later periods. Boys of noble households were initiated into their social roles through early apprenticeship. Historical records show that by the age of eleven many young noblemen served as "sublieutenants" with older and more experienced soldiers!

It was also a custom in the Middle Ages to indenture one's own children as domestic servants in other households, and to use other people's children as servants in one's house. This reflected several beliefs about education: that it is best done early, through imitation, and by strangers. "Waiting on people" was not regarded as debasing. The work of child servants was highly ritualized, with emphasis on forms of courtesy in language and behavior.

The sons of tradesmen were also sent away from home at an early age, to become apprentices to other tradesmen. The rationale was similar to that of the upper class, except of course that the sons of tradesmen had more practical things to learn than courtly manners. Thus medieval education reflected an image of childhood as a period for practical and independent functioning. What in present-day terms might seem to be a very demanding life for a child was not thought of as harmful. It was believed that early participation in the life of adults was natural and desirable.

> . . . Wherever people worked, and also wherever they amused themselves, even in taverns of ill repute, children were mingled with adults. In this way they learned the art of living from everyday contact. . . . In these circumstances, the child soon escaped from his own family, even if later he returned to it when he had grown up. (Ariès, 1962, p. 368.)

According to Philippe Ariès, an eminent French cultural historian who studied the evolution of the concept of childhood by synthesizing data from art, education, moral philosophy, pedagogy, economics, and literature, the present idea of childhood as a "special" period in life, one that is qualitatively different from adulthood, did not emerge in Europe until the seventeenth century. Ariès is careful to point out, however, that this development was not uniform across social classes; the nobility and the working classes were slower to change, and it was largely the growing middle class that created a "sentimental climate" around the idea of childhood. In historical terms, the seventeenth century is not further away than an instant in time. Therefore it is not surprising that some of Ariès' descriptions of middle class child-raising beliefs are still applicable today.

In Western Europe the seventeenth-century middle class parent responded to numerous educational and religious treatises that stressed the parents' responsibility for direct supervision over children. It was the religious moralists and pedagogues of the seventeenth century who convinced parents that children are not ready for life until they undergo a long period of grooming, care, purification, and training. They firmly believed that children are either sinners to begin with or eminently corruptible by bad influence. It was the parents' responsibility to insure the eventual salvation of their children by exercising vigilant control over their upbringing. These views created a new preoccupation with the physical, moral, and sexual problems of children, and more attention was focused on the *relationships* among members of the family, old and young, than ever before. Since there is ample evidence that it was the middle class that first organized itself around the idea of child-raising, the "connection between the concept of the family and the concept of class" is only too apparent. (Ariès, 1962, p. 414.)

By the eighteenth century the "retrieving" and protecting of the child from society at large was fairly well accomplished in the middle class, with the upper and lower classes to follow.[12] The responsibility for the health, education, morality, spiritual well-being, and afterlife of the child, particularly the middle class youth, was fully shifted onto his parents. The family, previously a loosely and more casually connected unit in vigorous commerce with the outside world, now drew its curtains and closed its doors to large parts of this world. It began to cultivate privacy and intimacy within the home. By the beginning of the nineteenth century the focus of family life was on the child. Nowhere was this more apparent than in colonial America.

Information about American child-raising beliefs and changing concepts of the nature of childhood reveals that during the period 1820–1860 American parents became increasingly interested in child-raising problems. Child-raising was considered an entirely rational process: specific methods could lead to specific results.[13] It was thought that *during the first six years of life the child's character was molded primarily by the mother.* Because she played a central role in determining the child's future well-being, the child-raising literature of the times called upon her

[12] Beliefs and values do run a cyclical course. When we read of a "new" theory advocating that education should be more "real" and more "revelant" or that children should "learn by doing" how "things really are," we should always consider the possibility that it is simply a reaction to a previous reaction. It appears that the eighteenth- and nineteenth-century parent might have gone too far in isolating his children from the world, and also too far in prolonging their economic and psychological dependence on the home.

[13] The material on American child-raising practices and beliefs presented in this section relies heavily on two papers: R. Sunley, "Early nineteenth-century literature on child-rearing," and M. Wolfenstein, "Fun morality: an analysis of recent American child-raising literature." Both papers as well as numerous others representing historical and cultural variations may be found in M. Mead and M. Wolfenstein (eds.), *Childhood in Contemporary Cultures* (Chicago: University of Chicago Press, 1963).

to control her own feelings and keep her thoughts pure! Consider the following quotation from a treatise written in 1849:

> Yes, mothers, in a certain sense, the destiny of a re-deemed world is put into your hands; it is for you to say, whether your children shall be respectable and happy here and prepared for a glorious immortality, or whether they shall dishonor you, and perhaps bring your grey hairs in sorrow to the grave, and sink down themselves at last to eternal despair. (Quoted in Mead and Wolfenstein, 1963, p. 152.)

Note that this emphasis on the first six years of life for char-acter formation and the elevation of the mother as the only one who had power over (and therefore responsibility for) the even-tual salvation or damnation of the child can hardly be attributed to the influence of Sigmund Freud. While his effect on American child-raising practices is indisputable, his ideas did not reach our shores until much later. (Freud lived from 1856 to 1939.)

The influence of the father on young children declined in nineteenth-century America. Functions previously assumed by him, such as disciplining the child and conducting daily religious observances, were gradually shifted to the mother. At the same time, schoolteaching emerged as an ideal occupation for unmar-ried women. Thus we can safely say that by the late nineteenth century the caretaking as well as educational functions of child-raising were completely shifted to women.

Social class differences were, of course, ever present. For ex-ample, wealthy women were more likely to bottle-feed their babies or to hire wet nurses than lower class mothers. It was be-lieved that poor women had a more ample supply of milk, and this in some way was thought to account for the lack of self-control among lower class children. It was thought that the mother's "ill-governed passions" might be transmitted through her milk!

It was also believed that babies should be "let to cry" in order to strengthen their lungs, convey to them the unacceptability of constant demands, and break their will. Mothers were thought virtuous if their children were toilet-trained at an early age. There is a record of a doctor who bestowed public praise upon a mother who "trained" her child at one month of age! To be clean was considered a sign of good morality; cleanliness was next to godliness. Sunley cites evidence to show that visitors from abroad noticed that Americans were personally very clean. Yet they also observed that an "interesting counterpart to this personal cleanliness was the untidy, unkempt appearance of the gardens, yards, streets, and sidewalks." (Quoted in Mead and Wolfenstein, 1963, p. 157.)

By far the most influential source of beliefs about children in the nineteenth century was the Calvinist doctrine of "infant depravity." According to this doctrine, the infant was certain to become a sinner unless he was carefully guided by his parents. Solitary prayer and Bible reading was recommended for young children. Masturbation was regarded as a mortal sin. Servants were viewed as the major source of moral corruption. In short, the infant was considered born "totally depraved" and eminently corruptible. He was by nature "bad." It was up to the parents to insure his salvation through grace.

As early as 1820 numerous Protestant sects—Methodists, Presbyterians, and Congregationalists—created groups known as maternal associations to exchange ideas about various techniques for breaking the will of the child and for achieving what was called "infant conversion." "Gentle drilling," isolation, and beatings were some of the techniques recommended for breaking the will. Discussion groups were set up to encourage and instruct mothers who might be too indulgent or "soft-hearted" and who therefore could not do their duty.

As the following description of infant conversion clearly illustrates, what was considered good and desirable behavior on the part of children at one time may today be seen as a sign of deep psychopathology:

> "Infant conversion" was considered highly desirable, for it meant that the child had reached the point of accepting *on its own* the truth of religion and hence was well on the road to being saved from depravity. There were many signs of such conversion—quick conversion not being considered as sound as the more gradual—among which signs were the practices of solitary prayer and Bible reading. . . . Little girls were apparently more often converted than boys, and the pages of the magazines contain quite a few melancholy stories of such children who became devoutly religious, submissive, seemingly drained of vitality and desires, and met an early death, often by the age of ten. Such children were held up as models of piety for the others. . . . (Mead and Wolfenstein, 1963, p. 160; italics added.)

Today, scarcely a hundred years later, we would think that a child who is "submissive, seemingly drained of vitality and desires," is very sick indeed. If this description pertained to a baby, a psychiatrist might suggest that the infant suffered from "marasmus," a form of infantile depression sometimes seen in babies who live in institutions where no one relates to them personally. A pediatrician might say that the child showed signs of the syndrome "failure to thrive," which is a general term covering just what the name implies. If such a description were applied to an older child, many clinicians would suggest the diagnosis "childhood schizophrenia." You will discover in the next chapter why.

At any event, it is clear that the image of the child underwent considerable change in America during the last century. However, Martha Wolfenstein, who studied American child-raising beliefs between 1914 and 1945, suggests that some of the changes are really only different expressions of the same preoccupation: How can we comfortably accept the reality of aggression and sexuality? She points out that while our specific attitudes and practices have changed, as a culture we are still uncertain about "whether what is enjoyable is not wicked or deleterious." She proposes that although we now allow children more direct impulse expression and more pleasure from their body, give them more attention, and in general believe in dovetailing with their wishes, we are still basically ambivalent about impulse expression. Wolfenstein interprets the data of child-raising literature to mean that instead of opposing, banishing, or condemning impulses, as in colonial days, we now attempt to deny their reality by diluting them. That is, by insisting that children are fun, that being a parent is fun, that parents should have fun with their children (or else what is wrong with parents?), that learning should be fun (or else what is wrong with teachers?), and that children should have fun being children (or else what is wrong with *them?*), we have embraced a new "fun morality," in which strict notions about good and evil are just as present as ever, only carefully disguised. Wolfenstein suggests that the concept of childhood and parenthood in terms of fun, pleasure, and play during the first half of our century and into the present may be an expression of a new Puritanism:

> Where formerly there was felt to be a danger that, in seeking fun, one might be carried away into the depths of wickedness, today there is a recognizable fear that one may not be able to let go sufficiently, that one may not have enough fun. . . . Fun and play have assumed a new obligatory aspect. . . . (Mead and Wolfenstein, 1963, p. 174.)

Indeed, the first half of this century was characterized by increased permissiveness toward children. There was the conviction that excessive interference with their desires would thwart their growth, but that left to their own devices children would "quit when they had enough." Even today, in child guidance clinics one often hears the same sad story. The child, now a patient, was not frustrated, not limited, not punished. He was given considerable freedom; his needs and demands were allowed free expression. How can it be that he is now completely unable to control himself and is the menace of his school and the terror of his neighborhood? Those who believe that the rebelliousness of today's youth is essentially destructive often blame Sigmund Freud and Benjamin Spock for their "effect" on child-raising practices and hold them responsible for what they judge to be lack of self-discipline, excessive willfulness, and untempered rebelliousness in young people.

Whatever one's opinion about these matters—and in the absence of data, one opinion is worth as much as another—it is important to realize that the upswing in permissiveness that characterized child-raising practices in the first half of this century must surely have been determined by more than the influence of one or two significant men.[14]

Emerging concepts of the child— a look into the future

We live today in a time when everything is changing rapidly, and beliefs, opinions, and convictions about the nature of children are hardly an exception. But today, as always, the parents of the parents exert considerable influence on the world of the

[14] Students with deeper interest in the effect of Freud upon the American public may refer to D. Shakow and D. Rapaport, *The Influence of Freud on American Psychology* (New York: International Universities Press, 1964).

child. Often, young parents vow never to repeat with their children the mistakes of their own parents. Or they decide that what was good enough for them will be good enough for their boys or girls. Through either rejection or acceptance, their point of departure is the previous generation. Consider the following statements by a contemporary mother regarding her attitudes and values toward raising her first-born child, a fourteen-month-old boy. She is a very young, highly articulate black woman. Her ideas about her baby telescope much from the past and contain some forecasts for the future:[15]

> . . . It's such a difference the way they brought me up and the way I would like to bring him up. . . . She's already set in her ways [referring to the baby's grandmother] and she can't change and actually come down to the understanding of how a child actually thinks, where I can, and this is the main problem right now. . . . Every time he falls down she runs to him, when he falls down, I stand and watch him. You know, I make sure it's nothing serious, and I know when he is just playing and when, you know, . . . really hurt, and I'll watch him, and he'll get up and I'll say "Now what happened to you?" and he'll start laughing and the tears will stop. But every time he falls, she'll run and pick him up. . . . We have carpet all over the floor; . . . he couldn't really hurt himself. . . . He's a very sloppy eater when he eats with her. I don't allow him to put his fingers all in his mouth and his hands all in the dish and so forth, and with her, . . . she allows him to do this.

[15] From the files of an ongoing research project on maternal stimulation and infant cognitive development conducted by Wells Goodrich, Mary Engel, William King, and Herbert Nechin at the City University of New York and the Montefiore Hospital and Medical Center (MH 17580–01).

The generational difference appears not only in relation to coddling, comforting, and babying but also in different methods of teaching the baby certain realities:

> I let him try anything once, you know, just to see what he is going to do, and I had an experience with him that actually taught him something, where I was trying to prove to my mother. . . . She would say, if you tell a child "hot" he'll leave it alone. And I said, well, how can he, if he doesn't know what "hot" is . . . if he touches it and feels the sensation. . . . So I said, well, I'll tell him "stop" again, and if he touches it, I'll say "hot." . . . So he goes up to . . . into the oven and comes back screaming, hollering, and crying, so I said "hot" and he'll leave it alone. I think that's the only way they know, because if they never felt hot, how do they know what hot is?

For a brief while, she and the baby lived in the house of the baby's father and the paternal grandparents. Here too the young mother consolidated her sense of difference from the previous generation. In discussing her husband's relationship with his mother, she said:

> . . . [His mother] more or less didn't give him any kind of supervision and if he pulled a tantrum, she wouldn't do anything about it, and she just let him, you know, have his way, and that's why I am so hard on him [the baby] now and my parents can't see that. Because I believe if you teach a child self-control from a very small age, they'll remember it. This is what his [her husband's] parents didn't. He wasn't taught at all. See, I really believe in self-control.

Yet she is not a restrictive mother. She chooses when she will be "hard on him" and when she considers freedom of action appropriate, and she takes strong steps to back up her convictions. This is how she explains her reasons for changing babysitters:

> [The new sitter] takes much better care of him with the other kids there. See, at the other place, she [the former sitter] didn't want him to do this, she didn't want him to do that. And you can't restrict a child that young! You have to give him the run of the house, or else you are the one that's caught up in the corner somewhere.

This same sensitivity to the limits of her influence and control over the baby comes through in her ideas about his future. When asked how far she would like her son to go in school, she explained:

> As far as he wants to go. 'Cause I don't believe that you can force anything on a child. I feel that they will accept you more if you respect their wishes also. I believe if you give a child respect, he'll give you respect. If he wants to go to college . . . I mean I would like for him to go, but if he doesn't want to go and he wants to take up something else, that's all well and good 'cause he has to live his life and I have to live mine.

This mother believes that character formation begins very early. She recognizes that by the age of fourteen months her baby has already learned complex patterns of communication, responds differently to various people, and learns best through direct experience. She has firm beliefs about the value of self-control as well as about the value of freedom. Her commitment to mutual respect, to the idea that babies will respect the mother to the degree that the mother respects them, is unusually modern. In fact, her array of convictions and beliefs gives a highly differ-

CHAPTER TWO

Diagnostic Aspects

Some general issues in diagnosis

Diagnosis or classification?

While doctors are quite sure that a diagnosis is indispensable to the prescription of treatment and is therefore a necessary step toward cure, psychologists or psychiatrists may hold any number of attitudes toward diagnosis. Indeed, the problems of identifying and understanding illness are quite different in medicine and psychopathology; the same word, *diagnosis,* obscures some essential differences important for us to understand.

Physicians have many advanced tests for diagnosing certain illnesses. Blood tests, urinalysis, and X-rays are only some of the methods by which symptoms are made *visible* and *countable.* Soon sophisticated computer techniques will be used to synthesize a great deal of information, from which physicians will be able to diagnose even the most complicated kinds of diseases. Psychologists are nowhere near attaining such precision, and it is possible that they will never even arrive at it. This might well be the case if the *dimensions of diagnosis* and the *factors in illness* in psychology turn out to be of quite a different order from those in medicine.

Let us consider one way in which diagnosis is different in medicine and in psychology. Suppose that a man is taken to a hospital with a very bad pain in the abdomen. Certain laboratory tests are performed and the physician decides that the *chances are* he has appendicitis. While there is never 100 percent certainty, the chances are very high, life is at stake, and the man is in severe pain. He is operated on that very night. When the appendix is exposed, it is indeed inflamed; the diagnosis is confirmed. Note that it is the operation—the treatment—that really confirms the diagnosis. The treatment informed the physician that his inferences were in fact correct.

Now consider an equally common diagnosis in psychology. A man goes to a clinic, where someone interviews him and writes down his complaints: he has periods of sleeplessness, he no longer enjoys his work, he has frequent fights with his wife, and his boss has recently told him that if he does not "shape up" he will soon lose his job. The man became worried about himself and that is why he came to the clinic for help. A psychiatrist "diagnoses" him as severely neurotic, somewhat depressed, and in a state of considerable panic. He is advised to enter psychotherapy, and after a year of interviews with a qualified psychologist or psychiatrist he feels better, his marriage is stabilized, and his boss no longer threatens to fire him. Was the treatment in any way a confirmation of the diagnosis? Maybe yes, maybe no. If you think about this example it will soon become clear that there might have been many factors working together that had nothing to do with the psychotherapy. Suppose the man's wife, who herself had felt somehow pent-up and chained to the household, obtained a job during this time. Eventually she became more cheerful, bought new clothes, did less housework—in short, she became a livelier and more interesting partner to him. Or suppose the man's boss experienced an upswing in business that made him less worried and therefore less demanding of his employees. One could list contingencies *ad infinitum,* and they would all be general in their effect and difficult to assess. It is far more difficult to ascertain the ultimate correctness of a psychological diagnosis by looking to the effect of treatment than the correctness of a medical diagnosis. *In medicine the effect of treatment is often the confirmation of the diagnosis; in psychology this is seldom the case.* It is important to remember these difficulties and to construct new models of diagnosis tailored to the realities of psychology as a science.

The life context of a patient is never irrelevant to diagnosing or curing him. But the context of mental illness bears a more complex role to symptoms than is the case in physical illness. In some psychological disturbances the context of the patient's life plays such a major role that a change in situation, or even in one aspect of the situation, can drastically redirect the course of the disturbance. Yet it is extremely difficult to contextualize the diagnosis of the illness—to ask, for example, "If this patient lived in such-and-such a context, would he also be ill?" There is really no answer to such questions at this time, yet everyone feels the need to take context into account in deciding how sick a mental patient is. Once psychotherapy has begun, the role of the patient's life context becomes clearer as the therapist gets to know the patient more and more.

Psychology, particularly clinical psychology, is a relatively new science. Thus it is not surprising that many clinicians themselves are confused by what it means to diagnose a patient. Rogers (1951), for example, feels that diagnosis serves only to retard the treatment; if a therapist knows that a patient he is seeing for the first time has been diagnosed as "schizophrenic," he will have a certain image of the person and will therefore never be able to transcend that generalization about his new patient. It is better, says Rogers, to dispense with diagnosis and to meet each new patient on his own terms, as a unique person. Other clinicians feel that without diagnosis they would just have to spend months of valuable time exploring and getting to know the patient; if a diagnosis had been made to begin with, they could have proceeded with certain forms of treatment right away. Both of these extreme positions have merit, and both contain mistakes in conceptualization.

The most frequent error in clinical psychology is mistaking classification for diagnosis. A label pinned on a person—such as "retarded," "neurotic," or "schizoid"—is never a diagnosis. Such labeling is nothing but classification. Strictly speaking, as anyone who has had a course in philosophy will agree, a person can never be classified; he can only be declared to belong to a group whose members share certain characteristics. For example, when we say that a child is "phobic," all we have said is that he exhibits characteristics like others who are so labeled. All we really know from this classification is that the child is unreasonably fearful, either of many things, as in a generalized phobia, or of some particular thing, such as flushing the toilet or going to school. Such a child may be different in significant ways from other children who are also called phobic. He may be more or less intelligent, he may have a good or poor relationship with his mother and father, he may be Roman Catholic, Protestant, or Jewish, and of course "he" may even be a girl! By classifying such a child as phobic, we set him aside from the rest of humanity to some degree—that is, we say that he is not like those who are *not* phobic—but such labeling is of little use when we ask ourselves what we can do to help him with his phobia. For that we need more than a classification; for that we need a diagnosis.

From the point of view of psychological functioning, labeling, or naming the group to which a person belongs, *implies and involves the possibilities of diagnosis.* To point to this as an error, however, is not to suggest that the problems of classification are irrelevant to psychopathology. With this distinction in mind, let us consider in turn some of the techniques of classification and diagnosis, with special emphasis on mental illness in children.[1]

Classification—the ambivalent game

There is no science without classification. Sciences differ in what they order and in how they create order from the infinite variety of phenomena in nature. Classification is so general in the sciences that there are even people who study *its* problems. These people, known as taxonomists, are the philosophers of classification who try to think of general rules for creating classes of phenomena. For example, George Gaylord Simpson is primarily an evolutionist, but he is also a taxonomist in that he has formulated some principles for creating classes that apply to sciences in general. (Simpson, 1961.)

Recent arguments among classifiers have a strong relativistic flavor. There has been a reexamination of an old yearning: to discover a "natural" classification scheme, uncontaminated by the perceptions of the scientist, that reflects an "inherent" order in nature. It is now understood that however much it may hurt, this yearning must be abandoned. The infinite variety of natural phenomena does not contain a secret scheme of things—whether animals with cleft hooves are to be grouped with only their own kind, with all mammals, or with all four-legged creatures is up to the classifier.

---

[1] Additional discussion of these issues may be found in M. Engel, "Dilemmas of classification and diagnosis," *Journal of Special Education,* 3 (1969), 231–39.

It has been suggested that all sciences that share the concerns of taxonomy—how classes should be constructed, what the rules for ordering nonevolutionary phenomena should be, and so on—should adopt multiple classification schemata, the utility of which is to be determined by their heuristic potential. If a new classification scheme directs us to look at the world in the same way as before, it is of no use. If it dictates or *teaches* a new perception of nature's order, let us use it, but not past the time of its novelty.

Class names make shorthand communication among scientists possible. If I want to save time I say, "This schizophrenic boy is not like a Kanner-type but more like a Mahler-type child." Such labels are convenient but they are also dangerous. In zoology, botany, and microbiology, where international communication among scientists takes place more often than among clinicians in mental health, it has been proposed that in addition to the multiple and peaceful coexistence of various classification schemata there should be an international scheme, again to insure ease of communication. (Simpson, 1961.)

But what of classification in clinical psychology and psychiatry? According to the medical historian Veith (1957), medical thinking was dominated by the Hippocratic influence until the eighteenth century, with the chief distinction in psychiatry being that of "chronic" and "acute." In the seventeenth century the proliferation of schemata began, with Sydenham's scheme of 2,400 different kinds of diseases. In the eighteenth century Pinel formulated five categories of insanity. The simplicity of this scheme derived from Pinel's pragmatism: he saw sense only in making those distinctions that resulted in different kinds of treatment for mental patients under his care. In contrast to the pragmatism of Pinel's scheme, Kraepelin's classification led to an overemphasis on the act of classifying itself, with a relative neglect of differences in treatment. Kraepelin's work had the advantage of setting psychiatry apart from neurology in that he proposed that some forms of mental illness could not be attributed to defects in the brain. But Kraepelin's classification was static and pessimistic with regard to prognosis.

Zigler and Philips (1961) have made an exhaustive review of all recent papers that are in any way critical of conventional psychiatric diagnoses. In their study Zigler and Philips note that the papers consistently confuse diagnosis with classification and conceptual schemata with labeling. They suggest that the failure of the Kraepelinian system was due not to the fact that symptoms are useless for classification but simply to the fact that they may not have been adequately ordered. Zigler and Philips make a strong plea for a reconsideration of the undesirability and lack of utility attributed to classification and for a differentiation of the questions concerning categorization of mental illness into those pertaining to classification schemata needed for research and schemata needed for treatment.

The reliability of a classification scheme should not be confused with its predictive validity. It is doubtful that perfect reliability would have much meaning; it is a profitable goal only for those who are interested in perfecting an existing classification scheme. Schemata are most fruitfully regarded as tools for discovery; questions concerning proper classification are likely to give rise to researchable hypotheses.

Szasz (1957) suggests that the very domain "psychiatric" is an ambiguous one and proposes an operational approach to psychiatric nosology. He lists the vast array of situations in which psychiatric diagnoses are made, such as veterans' hospitals, courts of law, child guidance clinics, and public schools. How, he asks, can one classification scheme be considered adequate for all these settings when the settings differ markedly in their methods of creating classes, as well as in the purposes for which the classes are created? To some people coal and diamonds are of the same class, but certainly not to the jeweler! Szasz suggests that the following psychiatric situations be distinguished on the American scene, with a distinct classification scheme developed for each: mental hospitals, private psychiatric practices, child guidance clinics, psychoanalytic training systems, military service, courts of law, and jails. One might add to this list schools and colleges as distinct psychiatric situations. Thus, like Simpson in zoology, Szasz calls for abandoning the search for a single, all-encompassing classification scheme in psychiatry.

There are thus general problems of classification that all scientists have to deal with: How are classes to be created? How can one test the usefulness of a classification scheme? There are also special problems of classification that pertain to individual sciences. In classifying mental illness, for example, one must sooner or later decide how to define a symptom, how to group symptoms, and which symptoms are really or only apparently different from others. Even within the field of mental illness there are very specific problems of classification, as, for example, in work with children. This is mainly because age does change the meaning of behavior. In working with children, the psychologist has to make developmental distinctions—for example, when the question arises as to whether some kinds of behavior are indeed "sick" or just "immature." Consider the case of speech problems. In very young children one could attribute inadequate or faulty speech to age or to a developmental lag. Either judgment implies that the child will outgrow his difficulty. But the same speech problem in an older child could be a sign of mental illness or of neurological malfunctioning, with the implication that waiting for the child to become older will not help. Developmental considerations affect the classification of a great many symptoms, such as bed-wetting, school phobia, and temper tantrums—in short, whenever problems of will and achievement are involved. For this reason, classification schemata that ignore developmental differences are of little help in working with children.

The recently completed report on classification by the Group for the Advancement of Psychiatry (1967) is a vast improvement over former schemata (Jenkins, 1964) in clinical work with children. This report marks the beginnings of multiple classification, insofar as the scheme provides independent assessment of symptoms and allows for the diagnosis of "normality." In addition, though its ten major categories of classification lean heavily on the 1961 Standard Nomenclature of Diseases, its concept of developmental deviations saves it from being a child-sized version of a classification scheme for adults. The authors of the GAP report recognize their inability to deal with sociocultural variations; however, other groups, such as committees of the American Orthopsychiatric Association, are taking steps toward making a systematic study of the diagnostic implications of sociocultural circumstances. (GAP, 1966.) Let us examine the classification scheme of the GAP report, which is likely to become widely used very soon.

The health-illness continuum in childhood

The authors of the GAP report found it sensible to classify mental health problems in children into the following ten categories, together with their respective subcategories:

1. Healthy Responses
   a. Developmental crisis
   b. Situational crisis
   c. Other responses
2. Reactive Disorders
3. Developmental Deviations
   a. Deviations in maturational patterns
   b. Deviations in specific dimensions of development
      (1) Motor
      (2) Sensory

      (3) Speech
      (4) Cognitive functions
      (5) Social development
      (6) Psychosexual
      (7) Affective
      (8) Integrative
    c. Other developmental deviations

4. Psychoneurotic Disorders
    a. Anxiety type
    b. Phobic type
    c. Conversion type
    d. Dissociative type
    e. Obsessive-compulsive type
    f. Depressive type
    g. Other psychoneurotic disorders

5. Personality Disorders
    a. Compulsive personality
    b. Hysterical
    c. Anxious
    d. Overly dependent
    e. Oppositional
    f. Overly inhibited
    g. Overly independent
    h. Isolated
    i. Mistrustful
    j. Tension-discharge disorders
      (1) Impulse-ridden personality
      (2) Neurotic personality disorder
    k. Sociosyntonic personality disorder
    l. Sexual deviation
    m. Other personality disorder

6. Psychotic Disorders
    a. Psychoses of infancy and early childhood
      (1) Early infantile autism
      (2) Interactional psychotic disorder
      (3) Other psychosis of infancy and early childhood

  b. Psychoses of later childhood
   (1) Schizophreniform psychotic disorder
   (2) Other psychosis of later childhood
  c. Psychoses of adolescence
   (1) Acute confusional state
   (2) Schizophrenic disorder, adult type
   (3) Other psychosis of adolescence
 7. Psychophysiologic Disorders
  a. Skin
  b. Musculoskeletal
  c. Respiratory
  d. Cardiovascular
  e. Hemic and lymphatic
  f. Gastrointestinal
  g. Genitourinary
  h. Endocrine
  i. Of nervous system
  j. Of organs of special sense
  k. Other psychophysiologic disorders
 8. Brain Syndromes
  a. Acute
  b. Chronic
 9. Mental Retardation
 10. Other Disorders (GAP, 1966.)[2]

Perhaps you imagine that each of these ten categories of psychological disturbance in childhood stands against a vast body of literature, a great deal of knowledge about diagnosis and cure.

---

[2] Students whose curiosity is excited by one or another of the ten psychopathological disorders (or their subcategories) proposed by the Group for the Advancement of Psychiatry may find additional discussions as well as further references in a number of books on mental illness in children. See, for example, J. W. Kessler, *Psychopathology of Childhood* (Englewood Cliffs, N.J.: Prentice-Hall, 1966), and Joint Commission on Mental Health of Children, *Crisis in Child Mental Health* (New York: Harper and Row, 1970).

Perhaps you also think that the number of children who suffer from each illness is known, and that if you only had enough time to read about them you would be able to acquire a comprehensive view of childhood mental illness. Nothing could be further from the truth.

The state of knowledge about child mental health is more like a map drawn after a flight over new terrain. While the map relies on some close-up shots, it is drawn primarily from photos taken from high above, giving only a bird's-eye view. The few close-ups that do exist were taken by people who have narrowed their interest to one kind of psychopathology, dealt for a long time with children suffering from one kind of disorder, and written about their efforts and experiences in depth. The bird's-eye shots were taken by people who conducted surveys, using questionnaires and high-powered statistics. The resulting map is uneven. Some parts of it are detailed, clear, accurate. Other parts of the map show only vaguely what the shape of the terrain might be. Thus our understanding of the psychopathology of childhood is not of the same quality over the various kinds of disturbances. In some people this fact creates irritation and impatience; in others it creates excitement and eagerness to do research.

Those who wish to understand the varieties of serious mental illness in children have to cope with considerable ambiguity in language. Such terms as *psychotic, schizophrenic,* and *autistic* are often used interchangeably because they have broad meanings and overlapping connotations. The following discussion will attempt to explain what is usually meant by psychotic. The distinction between schizophrenic and autistic (when it is observed) usually refers to a judgment that the child *became schizophrenic* after a certain period of time or that he *was autistic* from the beginning of his life. But this developmental distinction is not the only important one here, because the difference is also one of severity of illness. Autistic children are considered to be more deeply disturbed than schizophrenic youngsters. To complicate the matter of terminology even more, *autistic thinking* refers to very subjective, endogenous thinking which is not peculiar to the illness "autism," because some forms of autistic thinking also occur in schizophrenia.

In determining which of the many classes of emotional disorders in childhood should be included for detailed discussion in this section, I was not guided by considerations of incidence or prevalence.[3] Rather, in order to give neither an overstated picture of clarity nor one of confusion, I have chosen to discuss in detail *the area of psychotic disorders* followed by a consideration of *one of the psychoneurotic disorders.* Thus in the discussion of psychopathology that follows the student will have occasion to read about a puzzling kind of illness that has generated much disagreement. Following this, we will consider a circumscribed and fairly well-defined kind of disturbance.

Psychotic disorders of childhood

What is psychosis?

The GAP report defines psychotic disorders as involving severe disturbances in affect, perception, motility, speech, individuation, and thought. Let us briefly consider each of these processes and examine their implications for development.

Affect. Normal children have at their disposal a wide range of feeling states. They give evidence that they are capable of experiencing many different kinds of emotions. Most important, well-adjusted children feel and express emotions in a way that fits the situation or circumstance in which they find themselves.

[3] Incidence should not be confused with prevalence. The former means the rate at which new cases appear; the latter refers to the number of existing cases in a particular disease category.

Such children are said to be affectively "responsive," "flexible," and "appropriate."[4]

Children whose emotional growth is distorted often express their feelings in peculiar ways. Extreme examples are easy to draw. Think of a child of elementary school age who is afraid of specific objects—curtains, ironing boards, certain pieces of furniture—and in whom the sight of such objects will trigger a temper tantrum. Think of a first-grader who walks around saying "Good morning" to everyone when he enters the classroom and tells his classmates "I am so happy" while tears are running down his face.[5] Or think of a child whose elation comes and goes apparently without reason, whose affect of joy manifests itself at random times and in situations which seem not to give any cause for it. He can be as bewildering as a distressed child whose fear or anger cannot be explained or understood.

There are also children who show no feeling at all, who have withdrawn into themselves to such a degree that they appear to vegetate emotionally. Finally, there are children whose behavior appears quite usual for the most part but who occasionally give vent to an excess of rage from which they cannot be coaxed and in which they seem out of reach.

Such disorders of affect can become quite extreme. They are an earmark of psychosis. However, the clinician must always take care to base such a judgment on ample data! Note that all these examples illustrate affective display (or withholding of feeling) that seems very unwarranted. Since children can seldom explain their own behavior (the common parental injunction "*Why* do you do things like that?" seldom brings a clear answer), the adult is left to find the reason for the child's conduct. The affective dis-

---

[4] These words are set off in quotation marks because in the vocabulary of the clinical psychologist they have special connotations acquired through use and, like jargon or idioms, are difficult to define.

[5] I am indebted to Dr. David Reiser of Boston for this example.

turbance of very ill children leaves even the professionally trained observer confused and at a loss to answer the "why."

Perception. For experimental psychologists, the term *perception* means "giving meaning" to sensation. Through interpreting what we experience in the auditory, tactual, and visual modalities we build up an image of the world that corresponds, more or less, to that of others around us. There are many reasons why children might have perceptual problems. They need not necessarily have a serious emotional disturbance. For example, it is not unusual for children to have trouble distinguishing the letters *b* and *p,* because these letters have a certain perceptual similarity. However, the perceptual difficulties of psychotic children are much more severe, leading them to make gross misinterpretations of stimuli. An extreme example is that of a child who hears or sees things that no one else hears or sees. Psychologists often say that such a child hallucinates. It is not just that he *imagines* the presence of stimuli that do not exist; he also *sees* or *hears* them. Such children often confuse time and space aspects of the world. In lesser degrees of illness they sometimes sufficiently distort what they see or hear to become disoriented with regard to where they are and to what is happening to them. Because perceptual difficulties are also present in brain-damaged children, it is often very hard to differentiate between organically damaged children and those who are seriously mentally ill.

Motility. Psychotic children often show peculiar mannerisms of movement which seem to have a repetitious and driven quality. Compulsive finger-twiddling is often observed in psychotic children, as are head-banging and other forms of self-stimulation and self-injury. Such children may also have peculiarities in gait and posture. As with perceptual problems, aberrations in motility confuse the diagnostic picture when we try to differentiate between organically damaged and psychotic children.

Speech. Some psychotic children are mute—that is, they do not speak at all; or they may hum or make odd noises that seem to have no communication value. Such children are frequently called "autistic." Mutism is only one of many forms of speech peculiarities from which clinicians try to infer the degree of disturbance in individuation and thought, the next two processes to be discussed.

Individuation. In normal development, children move away from the mother, begin "cruising" around on the floor, and develop an interest in the external world. Some psychotic children, however, remain "fused" with the mother, tied to her emotionally and in space. They cling to her and become terrified when they feel she might leave the room. Still others remain confused about their body parts and may mistake another's hand or foot for their own. This shows that they have never acquired a sense of their own body as separate from that of others. Problems of individuation also appear in the confusion of "I" with "you" in speech and in the tendency to refer to oneself in the third-person singular.

Of course, some confusion about the separateness of self exists even in normal life. *Think* about the shoe on your foot! You suddenly become very aware of it being a shoe *on* your foot. But ordinarily, and if it is a comfortable shoe, you do not maintain a sense of separateness between the shoe and your foot any more than you remain constantly aware that your wristwatch or your eyeglasses are not part of your body. Such special "loss of boundary" is normal. In the case of psychotic children, this kind of fusion exists with many things and people and shows a general inability to experience oneself as separate.

Thought. The thought processes of psychotic children are available to be analyzed if the children talk or write; otherwise clinicians have to infer everything from their behavior, which is a very difficult thing to do. Primitive and peculiar are the two characteristic features of the thought processes of psychotic children. These characteristics of thought gain many kinds of expression. Psychotic children often seem not to have any control over their thinking. Some openly complain that there are thoughts that "happen" to them and that they occasionally wish to be rid of. Their thinking is often replete with frightening images. Their ideas are loosely connected, and they often jump from one idea to another. Logical sequence, even in the most minimal form, is often absent; and there may be a unique symbolism attached to certain thoughts. These children may have a passionate investment in some topics about which they might know a great deal, yet they may be unable to solve the simplest of problems on the level of thought.

It is very difficult to separate problems of thought from other aspects of illness because thoughts are such a major avenue for the expression of anxiety, fear, and apprehension. It is certainly unwise to separate thought from feelings except for the purposes of a discussion concerning various aspects of mental illness.

It goes without saying that in assessing the seriousness of disturbance in the various processes just discussed the clinician must always take the child's age into account. Certain forms of primitive behavior are less serious at some ages than at others; clinicians must always try to distinguish between "immaturity" and "psychopathology."

With these brief introductory remarks about the definition of psychosis in the GAP report, let us now consider in detail some major theorists in the field of psychotic disorders in childhood.

Bettelheim's theory of childhood psychosis

The Orthogenic School at the University of Chicago was created by Dr. Bruno Bettelheim for the treatment of autistic children. Here, in a protected residential and carefully planned physical setting, autistic and psychotic children receive around-the-clock care for long periods of time. Some children go to the Orthogenic School when still in early childhood and stay until they are ready to enter an occupation or college. Generally, the parents are not involved in the treatment; rather the children are "given over" for a time to the staff of the school. This feature of the treatment has aroused much controversy in clinical circles; it is more typical to work closely with parents while children are being treated for psychological disturbance.[6]

Bettelheim sees autism as a desperate and determined attempt to blot out stimuli in order to avoid pain and disappointment. Autistic children have "quelled the impulse to act." Having terminated all commerce with the external world, autistic children have found a way to ward off the possibility of further hurt. Autism is the last fortress, a single, massive defense against pain. It is an "empty fortress" because it is no longer enriched by "a dialogue with reality." Convinced by early traumatic experiences that the external world is not responsive to their needs, autistic children have given up all efforts to have an effect on the world. They have ceased acting on their own behalf. They have stopped willing. Those who refuse to talk give the most eloquent testimony of their total withdrawal from action. After all, one cannot talk without at least the implication of interchange with the world.

The following discussion will examine two foci of Bettelheim's thinking: critical periods for the development of autism and degrees of autistic withdrawal. Such ideas enrich our understanding of this mysterious illness and enliven our thinking about a group

[6] Bettelheim's philosophy of treatment and his formulation of the origins of the illness of autism are set down in detail in *The Empty Fortress* (New York: Free Press, 1967). This book contains some of the most beautifully written case histories of autistic children available. These studies are the bulk of the book, and any attempt to summarize them here would do them an injustice.

of youngsters for whom the joy of life is often lost before it has begun.

The concept of critical periods has its origins in ethology. Through the studies of Lorenz, Tinbergen, Hinde, Sluckin, and others, we have become aware that among animals certain forms of behavior must be acquired during a critical period or they will not be acquired at all. For example, a chick will follow its mother only if it had a chance to do so when it was very young; if it is confronted with its mother after this period has passed, the chick will show indifference to the hen. (Sluckin, 1965.) Thus the events, or environmental givens, at a specific time in development may determine the animal's future behavior to a large extent.

The concept of critical periods has to be used in a much broader sense in relation to human behavior. Here it is best to think in terms of "periods of heightened sensitivity." (Hinde, 1963.) For example, while it is much easier to learn a second language early in life than in adulthood, this does not mean that a second language can be acquired only in childhood. Even now you can decide to learn to play the violin or the cello. You may become quite a good player. But it is unlikely that having begun to play in young adulthood, you will ever perform in Carnegie Hall.

With respect to the development of personality, of interest in human relationships and investment in the world, Bettelheim reaches the conclusion that there are at least three periods *in the first two years of life* that are critical for the development of autism. The illness may originate (1) in the first six months of life, when people are still not differentiated in the baby's experience; (2) between six and nine months of age, when "people" should become "persons"; and (3) between eighteen months and two years of age, when the child should learn that he can have an effect on the environment and an interchange with the world. The child learns to walk, to talk, and to control his bowels, and in all these ways he can learn that he has a *will*. Should the child during any one of these periods receive the message that the world is frustrating, unresponsive, and irrelevant to his needs, he may "conclude" that there is no point in trying to relate to such a frustrating world. Unless he has already experienced himself as able to have an effect on the world and occasionally to mold it to his wishes, when his needs are frustrated he is left unprotected against the conclusion that the entire world is unresponsive and insensitive to him. Undesirable consequences of the infant's efforts to contact the world are more critical for the development of autism if they occur before the second year of life —that is, before he could have the feeling that he is able to interact with the human environment.

It should be noted that by a frustrating or insensitive environment Bettelheim does not mean obvious neglect. Many autistic children have been well cared for physically during infancy. Rather he means a combination of circumstances and events from which the child can "conclude" that although the environment will take care of him it will do so on its own terms only, and that he, the infant, cannot have any communication with it. The child senses that he is not really treasured, and no amount of physical caretaking on the part of his parents can mask their basic rejection of his existence. Thus the autistic child develops without the ability to even imagine a satisfying world. His inner life is an empty fortress.

Bettelheim recognizes three degrees of autism, depending upon the severity of the early experiences just described. First, there are the mute autistic children, who have no interest in any part of the outside world. Their failure to speak is one manifestation of their total withdrawal and lack of investment in anyone or anything. When one is with such a child one often feels like a "thing"; one feels totally ignored by the child, as though one did not exist. The withdrawal is complete. Second, there are autistic children who do talk and who have occasional angry outbursts.

Through these communications they show that they have some inner life, however undeveloped. Still, such children do not "act on their own behalf" and have no connectedness with other people. Finally, there are autistic children whom clinicians often call "schizophrenic." These children are the least affected and have the best prognosis. They often have a richer inner life; their fantasies are charged with a sense of reality. They are really engaged in a desperate struggle with a world that they experience as hostile and very powerful. While these children also do not form relationships with others in the usual sense, they do express their feelings and thoughts, and therefore those who are trained to understand their chaotic behavior can often decode their complicated messages.

Des Lauriers' theory of childhood schizophrenia

Des Lauriers' explanation of childhood schizophrenia departs from most psychoanalytic formulations. It is also different from that offered by Bettelheim. Des Lauriers believes that the schizophrenic has not withdrawn from the world; rather

> he is essentially an individual who has lost the capacity to experience himself as real. . . . His total behavior would have to be understood . . . not as a defense against a threatening world, or as an escape from unbearable experiences, but as a disorganized and frantic effort at discovering or rediscovering himself, at establishing the bounds and limits of his reality. . . . (Des Lauriers, 1962, p. 51.)

For Des Lauriers, the psychological existence of the individual depends upon his inner sense of individuality, his ability to "know" the psychological and physical boundaries that differentiate one person from another. One can "know" and "feel" the reality of oneself only by experiencing oneself *in contrast* to others. Freud also believed this to be true. But Des Lauriers departs from Freud in his belief that the problems the schizophrenic deals with are not the ones that caused his illness. These are the special problems of *being schizophrenic now*. Thus there is no point in interpreting to the patient the reasons for his behavior, and there is little reason to try to unravel *ex post facto* what happened to make the patient sick. Whereas the more conventional therapist would try to decode the chaotic messages relayed in the patient's language and behavior, Des Lauriers assumes that there is no order in the chaos, no message in the confusion. The chaos and confusion *are* the illness. The work of the therapist is to replace them with an order and clarity relevant to the present life of the patient. Des Lauriers compares the schizophrenic process to an orchestra without a conductor or a score. Every member of the orchestra is playing something, but until there is a common score or a conductor there can be no melody, no music; there can only be noise. So it is with the schizophrenic. He can think, often talk, eat, sleep, and "behave" in many different ways; but these behaviors and the psychological processes underlying them are not "orchestrated," so the patient is confused and deeply frightened by his illness.

It is a fact of the human condition that the ultimate pleasure is in giving and receiving—in interacting with others. This interaction is predicated on a sense of separateness. A person cannot love someone unless he has a concept of some "other" who is not himself. The ultimate terror resides in a loss of self, an absence of separateness, a loss of the sense of reality. According to Des Lauriers, this sense of unreality is the kernel of schizophrenia. Against this the patient struggles, trying to find firm footing in time and space and in a sense of his own reality. But for reasons that Des Lauriers recognizes as developmental, the patient is not able to find firm footing. Let us then, he says, ignore what made him sick. Let us show little or no interest in his "crazy" behavior. It has no meaning any more. Instead, Des Lauriers suggests that the therapist become "an insistent presence" in the child's life, impressing on him in every possible way simple and indisputable facts about reality and teaching him, as it were, where his body begins and ends, the facts of physical pleasure and pain, the boundaries of time—an hour, a day, a week—and the boundaries of the space in which he finds himself. The therapist must not allow the patient to "abstract" himself from any situation. There should be no validation of any kind of unreal fantasies. By insisting that the patient become *real*, by gentle but relentless emphasis on the simplest realities of living, the therapist gradually leads the patient out of psychosis.

Goldfarb's empirical approach to schizophrenia

The staff of the Ittelson Center for Child Research has for some time devoted itself to the investigation of the nature of childhood schizophrenia. The writings of William Goldfarb and his colleagues stand as excellent examples of empirical research on the causes of schizophrenia and of ways in which research results may lead to new approaches in clinical management. (Goldfarb, 1961; Goldfarb, Mintz, and Stroock, 1969.)

The point of departure for the work at the Ittelson Center is the assumption that any group of children diagnosed as schizophrenic comprises youngsters with a variety of symptoms and causes of these symptoms. Thus treatment is addressed primarily to specific deficiencies in the adaptive skills of each child. But attention is also given to "corrective socialization," because in all cases "the environment has failed to meet [the child's] requirements for being able to perceive reality, to orient himself to it, to organize it in his own mind, and to manipulate it effectively." (Goldfarb, Mintz, and Stroock, 1969, p. 7.)

The most striking feature of the behavior of schizophrenic children is their complete puzzlement with the world, a confusion that reflects their parents' bewilderment, uncertainty, and passivity toward them. Goldfarb and his colleagues have long recognized the importance of clarifying the obvious question of differential diagnosis: Could some of the puzzlement of the children, as well as their incapacity to organize perceptual and cognitive materials, be due to organic deficiencies such as brain damage?

It should be noted that there are few writers and clinicians working with schizophrenic and autistic children who discard the possibility that this devastating mental illness is at least in part organically determined. Some, like Bender (1953), see in childhood schizophrenia a very clear expression of organic damage and have built their theories on the assumption that brain damage is the major determinant of schizophrenia. Others, like Bettelheim (1967), find the assumption of organic etiology unnecessary and are able to give an entirely psychological explanation of the illness.

Goldfarb's research is mentioned here as an example of an empirical contribution to illuminating the problem of etiology in childhood schizophrenia. Empirical research of this sort is very rare in clinical work. Most clinicians use case reports and personal observations as tools for evaluating evidence much more often than data collected by less personal means, for they consider the more commonly used techniques of psychological research (questionnaires, tests, recorded behavioral observations) too cumbersome and not sufficiently sensitive. They generally regard methods used in personal participation with the patient as more promising for unraveling clinical mysteries. It is for this reason that Goldfarb's work is unique.

For the purposes of his research, Goldfarb defined childhood schizophrenia as a "behavior disorder characterized by many and qualitatively serious defects of the ego." (Goldfarb, 1961, p. 10.) He focused on three kinds of defects that he repeatedly observed in children being treated at the Ittelson Center: (1) absence of pleasure in overt behavior and thus absence of the integrating force that pleasure will bring to an activity, (2) preferences for proximal (touch, taste, smell) over distance (hearing, seeing) receptors, and (3) deviant speech. Two kinds of etiology were considered: intrinsic problems of capacity and extrinsic problems of social experience and motivation. This distinction was based on the fact that some children "looked like" brain-damaged children with a poor physical start in life and specific organic inabilities, whereas other children seemed "normal" in their physical development while their environment seemed sufficiently inadequate to account for their disturbed and often bizarre behavior. But whatever *the* cause, it was clear that parental perplexity, bewilderment, and confusion were present in a majority of these cases, and it made sense to think of this as a major determinant of the deviance in the children—whether the parents' perplexity arose for reasons of their own personality or because indeed they produced a bewildering and confusing baby.

Goldfarb proposed that the relative importance of environmental and organic causes could be better evaluated if several groups of children were compared in some "objective" way. His work began with twenty-six children diagnosed as schizophrenic at the Ittelson Center. The group consisted of eighteen boys and eight girls between the ages of six and a half and eleven who had been in psychotherapy for periods ranging from two to forty-one months. These children were compared with twenty-six schoolchildren who served as a control group. The latter group of children had no known psychological disturbances and matched the patient group on several relevant variables, such as age, sex, and social class.

The Ittelson Center does not accept children with obvious

and serious brain damage; it takes only those with doubtful signs of organicity. Yet after ordinary examination by psychiatrists, sixteen of the twenty-six schizophrenic youngsters were classified as organically damaged, while ten were seen as organically intact. These diagnoses were made before the experimental tests were given and were based solely on the psychiatrists' intuitive understanding of the effects of brain damage on behavior.

From the results of these examinations all the children in the study were categorized as either normal, organically damaged schizophrenic, or organically intact schizophrenic. Then an extensive battery of tests was administered to them and careful observations were made for the purpose of rating qualitative aspects of behavior. Home visits were also set up, during which trained observers rated each youngster's family on a number of dimensions of interaction. Comparisons were then made between the three groups of children in order to find out what aspects of deficiency characterized each group.

A summary of results showed that there were no differences among the three groups in measures such as height, weight, auditory and visual acuity, color vision, and lateral dominance of eye, foot, or hand. Several tests did differentiate between all normal and all schizophrenic children, though not between schizophrenic children judged to be organically damaged and those judged to be organically intact. Such measures can thus properly be called *tests of psychosis*. These tests—including ratings of adequacy of attention span, ability to sustain effort, degree of restlessness, superiority of muscle tone, superiority of speech patterns, and several more obviously neurological measures (finger-to-nose test)—showed schizophrenic children to function worse than normal children.

Finally, a number of tests distinguished among all three groups and were thus identified as *tests of organicity*. The Rail-walking Test, the Wechsler Intelligence Scale for Children, Raven's Progressive Matrices (a nonverbal intelligence test), and the Lincoln-Oseretsky Test (a measure of motor adequacy) are examples of the tests that set apart the organically damaged group from all others.

Specially trained neurologists were then asked to examine the children. For this purpose the group was enlarged to include youngsters with behavioral disorders, in order to stack the cards against the tendency to overlabel schizophrenic children as brain damaged. (If only normal and schizophrenic children had been examined by the neurologists, they could have judged from the unruly behavior of some of the children which ones were likely to be schizophrenic and which ones were likely to be in the normal group. The children with behavioral disturbances were included in order to "confuse" the neurologists.) The degree of agreement between the neurologists' assessments of brain-damaged schizophrenic children and the earlier assessments of the psychiatrists was 81 percent, showing a high correspondence between the intuitive judgment of psychiatrists and the results of neurological examination. These results suggest that tests as well as clinical judgments can and do differentiate between schizophrenic children who are and are not organically damaged. Thus it is now clear that the usual clinician's dilemma—"Is this child brain damaged *or* schizophrenic?"—is relative nonsense; a child can be either or both.

Perhaps the most interesting feature of Goldfarb's research was the home observations. Trained observers made three one-hour visits to each home, attempting to include mealtime, in order to rate the interactions of family members. Various members were rated on forty-six seven-point scales, with a high rating reflecting adequacy of functioning. The home observers were not informed of the original classification of the child. When their ratings were summarized, the families of normal children emerged as most adequate, those of organic schizophrenic children as next most adequate, and the families of nonorganic schizophrenic children as least adequate. This again shows the value of the distinction between the three groups and leads us to believe in the multiple etiology of this illness.

Mahler's theory of symbiotic psychosis

It was not until 1940 that adult psychiatry began to accept the existence of the condition now known as "early infantile autism," an illness described several years earlier by Dr. Leo Kanner. By the mid-1940's Margaret Mahler had collected several cases of psychosis in childhood and was beginning to demonstrate that her cases were remarkably different from Kanner's autistic children yet clearly cases of psychosis. During the 1950's Dr. Mahler formulated her theory of "symbiotic psychosis." Today she is advancing a rather comprehensive *developmental theory* built on the assumption of the inevitable necessity of relationships with important people during the first two years of life. Through her studies of children whose psychological development had obviously gone awry, Mahler arrived at some general developmental formulations regarding changes in the human condition during infancy. (Mahler, 1968.)

Whereas the autistic child has achieved the state of supreme separateness described by Kanner, and has barricaded himself in "the empty fortress" so richly described by Bettelheim, the symbiotically psychotic child has never achieved a sense of "me-ness," a sense of himself as a separate individual. Even in normal life, of course, the sense of separateness is occasionally lost. When one is in love or feels very close to another, it is easy to feel as though one is part of that other person. Life is punctuated with such experiences of symbiosis. But these experiences are departures from the usual sense of self, from the customary inner conviction that one is an individual with separate feelings, sensations, and thoughts.

In symbiotically psychotic children the possibility of separate experience does not exist. They act as though their very survival depended on close physical proximity to the mother. Psychologically speaking, these children are part of the mother, an aspect of her; they exist in her and through her. They give evidence of serious disturbances in perception of body image and in body functioning and they often obviously confuse themselves with other people. When one such child was given a test which required him to place wooden blocks into their appropriate slots, he took the psychologist's hand and made it do all the work, thus confusing his own hand with that of the other person. Another child, whose mother was expecting a new baby, often started the day vomiting, saying that there was a baby in *his* tummy that made him have to throw up.

What might be the etiology of symbiotic psychosis in children? Mahler reminds us that the intrauterine parasite-host relationship between the mother and the baby must continue for a while after birth. This is because the human infant is completely helpless and entirely dependent on his mother (or on whoever mothers him) for survival. After birth, a kind of "social symbiosis" replaces the intrauterine condition; a psychological unity is established between mother and baby. In addition to being completely dependent on the mother for survival, the infant of course cannot make his needs known in words. This fact underlines the indispensability of the symbiotic unity that continues in this "social" sense after the biological unity has been dissolved.

How is it possible for the mother to "know" when the baby is in discomfort, when he has had enough food, stimulation, or wakefulness, when he is "just tired," or when he does not "act right"? Mahler's assumption is that the mother remains in a state of sensitive empathy with the child; the child in turn "learns" that his distress will be understood and that something will be done to make him comfortable. He learns that if he is in need, this will not last forever, that someone will be there to change him, feed him, and protect him.

The growing years may be regarded as the span of time during which the child learns to know reality—how things are, what makes them work, how events are ordered. Thus the social symbiosis immediately after birth is the infant's first "lesson" in reality. It is assumed that if caretaking is insensitive, erratic, and lacking in empathy, the baby will not learn reality; rather he will continue to flail about with his needs and search, increasingly ineffectually, for a stable and satisfying state of affairs. But if caretaking is adequate, sensitive, empathic, and predictable, the baby will "use" it in developing a psychological sense of external reality. According to Mahler, it is erroneous to speak of psychotic children as having become alienated from reality; rather they have "never attained a solid sense of external reality." (Mahler, 1968, p. 47.)

Mahler is intent on clarifying her assumption that separation from the mother in infancy, by itself and in and for itself, cannot account for psychosis in children. She maintains that babies are incredibly hardy, resilient, and responsive to care, even if that care does not come from their natural mother. To support this point Mahler cites research about the psychological development of children born in concentration camps whose mothers were killed and who later developed fairly well (free of psychosis).

With respect to the "nature-nurture" controversy in the etiology of schizophrenia, Mahler explains that very sturdy infants may become psychotic under the impact of critically timed and devastating experiences in their infancy. For those babies who are very vulnerable constitutionally, "normal mothering" may prove insufficient in meeting their special requirements for extreme degrees of protectiveness and participation in the symbiotic partnership on the part of the mother.

Mahler's ideas about infantile development play an important part in her theory about the way in which inadequate symbiotic participation in early life can lead to a total inability to separate from the mother and to develop a sense of self.

According to Mahler, the first month of life is a period of "normal autism." External reality has no separate meaning, there is no sense of self, and the baby is in a state of "primitive hallucinatory disorientation." His main "purpose" is to maintain a primitive state of homeostasis. The person who insures this is interchangeable. That is, it seems to matter little to the infant who ministers to his needs, who relieves him of his distress.

At the end of the first month a maturational crisis seems to take place; it can be shown that the baby's overall physiological sensitivity to external stimuli increases at this time. This point marks the beginning of a long and gradual process of psychological separation from the mother, the beginning of individuation. Now the symbiotic phase begins. It culminates in the fourth or fifth month of life. During this phase the baby becomes increasingly aware of people as specific and distinct. By the end of the symbiotic phase the infant is able to discriminate facial expressions and strangers; "nonmothers" are subjected to "customs inspection," which is a typical steady stare into the face of the stranger as though studying the facial properties of the other.

If during this time the baby has had adequate symbiotic caretaking, he will, at around five months of age, develop a great interest in matters not pertaining to the mother. If the symbiotic needs have not been met, the baby cannot move out, psychologically speaking, and therefore his emerging sense of self will be seriously impaired. Normally, though, there is at this time a "second hatching," a physical turning away when held on a lap, a visual turning elsewhere for stimuli.

Between ten and sixteen months of age the infant reaches the peak of the "hatching period." He discovers that he can move, crawl, creep, displace himself in space at his own will. He begins to explore and to "practice" his new-found skills. His explorations are often interrupted by a quick and obvious return to the mother, for "emotional refueling": "She is still there, I am still safe and watched over, I can go out again and explore some more!" As the infant gradually discovers what he can do, how far he can go, and what is outside his immediate line of vision, he also finds out who he is and where his place is in the general scheme of things. But he still needs someone to return to, someone who will scoop him up, comfort him, and take care of him between his journeys. Otherwise he might not venture out so readily.

By eighteen months of age the child reaches the peak of the "practicing period." He is joyously engaged in ever newer ventures, examining things, taking objects into his hands and his mouth, looking, feeling, testing. His behavior suggests that he feels very strong, very able, very powerful, very much himself.

Note that in addition to a satisfactory symbiotic phase, further guarantee of individuation comes from the maturational push for motility. That is, developmental forces propel the child to use his large muscles. Should the quality of his relationship to his mother bind him to her, in the sense of a symbiotic tie, he can be expected to suffer anxiety pertaining to the most intense conflict, that between his wish to stay merged with her and his maturational need to exercise his independence. It is easy to see how such a conflict, unbearable enough in its adult versions, might shatter the psychological development of a child under two years of age.

It is important to note that not everyone would agree with all of Mahler's formulations of normal infantile development. There is still room for a good deal of research on the exact nature and timing of some of the major developmental events of the first two years of life.

Very little has been said thus far about the mother's role in the evolution of psychosis. The notion of the "schizophrenogenic mother"—that is, the mother who induces schizophrenia—was popular for a while in clinical circles, but it gave way to a more refined understanding of the interaction between temperamental characteristics of babies and personality factors in their mothers. Today it is more usual to talk of good and poor "matches" in mother-infant pairs, rather than to blame mothers for it all.

Of course, every clinician is always ready to offer numerous examples of destructive mothering. I cannot help recalling a case involving a three-year-old symbiotically psychotic patient, a little girl, whose mother wished to have her cured. The baby would not allow the mother out of her sight. The mother could not even go out of the room without the baby screaming! The baby was becoming heavy to carry. The mother wished to have more children but felt that she could not, since every time she moved away from this one the child yelled, cried, protested, and had a temper tantrum. The mother's mobility was severely restricted and her role as a wife had deteriorated completely.

The pair was taken on in treatment. For several weeks the little girl nestled in her mother's lap while I quietly played with some toys at the other end of the room. After a while, the child ventured off her mother's lap and craned her neck to see what I was doing. After six months she began to come over and finger some of the toys, only to run back to her mother as though she had touched something hot or seen something awful. All this time the mother sat completely passive, watching, giving tacit consent. (How tempting it was to push the process, to cajole her to come over, to praise her for her adventuresomeness. I refrained from this. It was very much like squirrel-taming on a park bench.)

By the end of a year the child seemed sufficiently reassured to spend the entire therapy hour in silent play with me while her mother sat at the other end of the room watching us. I was beginning to believe that, given another few months, she might allow the mother out of the room. But after the child had had several sessions of play with me, I received a telephone call from the mother. She said that she had decided her daughter was now much improved and that she felt sure the rest would go well without treatment. She was terminating therapy.

The moral of the story is not hard to tell. The mother could not tolerate the child's growing independence—such as it was—demonstrating the two-way nature of the symbiotic tie. The intolerance of some parents of improvement in their children is a reality known to every clinician at least as well as the uncompromising determination of other parents to see their child well.

Psychoneurotic disorders of childhood

The GAP report approaches psychotic disorders of childhood developmentally, separating early infantile autism from psychoses in later childhood and adolescence. Its schema for the classification of neuroses, however, is not constructed along developmental lines. For while there is general agreement that neuroses originate in childhood, too many questions must still be answered before firm conclusions can be drawn. For example, it is not known why certain children "choose" one kind of neurosis over another, or why some children mirror the neuroses of their parents while others seem beset with personality problems directly opposite to those of their parents. It is also not known whether, given the "choice" of one type of neurosis early in life, there is a predictable course to its evolution in adulthood.

The younger the child, the harder it is to predict his future mental health status, for the organization of the young child's personality is extremely fluid. The earlier in life a child is diagnosed, the more likely it is that his circumstances will change. Finally, in general the younger the child, the younger (and more malleable) his parents. Psychologists do not know the relative weight of various external factors in the evolution of neuroses. One must always guard against making complex generalizations for large groups of children. But it is possible for clinicians to gain considerable understanding of the neurotic difficulties of particular children about whom there is a good deal of information. The explanatory work of the clinician in formulating a diagnosis is different from the predictive work of the researcher. The researcher has relatively little information about a large number of people, whereas the clinician works with a great deal of information about a limited number of patients.[7]

The following discussion of psychoneurotic disorders in children is intended to give an overall view of *some major ideas* pertaining to the origin and structure of neuroses. The usefulness of these ideas will then be demonstrated by a clinical case of a boy with an obsessive-compulsive neurosis. Note the consideration of neuroses does not call for examination of a number of separate theories, as was the case in the discussion of psychotic disorders. The major ideas of psychoneurosis are all variants of Freud's formulations; theories that parade as "new" are really elaborations and adaptations of Freud's thinking.

What is neurosis?

After presenting a rather brief definition of psychoneurotic disorders, in which we are reminded that neuroses are *uncon-*

[7] This difference between the clinician and the researcher in the kind of information used and in the manner of working with it gives rise to much disagreement about the nature of various kinds of illness. Epistemologists, those who study the ways in which we gather information and weave it together, have recently turned their attention to epistemological problems in psychology. Both philosophically minded psychologists and psychologically minded philosophers have found the difference between prediction and explanation of great interest. See, for example, A. Kaplan, *The Conduct of Inquiry* (San Francisco: Chandler, 1964); M. Sherwood, *The Logic of Explanation in Psychoanalysis* (New York: Academic Press, 1969).

scious and habitual ways of dealing with anxiety, the authors of the GAP report briefly characterize several types of neuroses: phobic, conversion, depressive, obsessive-compulsive, as well as mixtures of these. The definitions are brief because they are written not to teach but to define and give common ground to those understandings that most clinicians spend many years acquiring.

Let us dissect the terse definitions of the GAP report and examine several aspects of the psychoanalytic theory of neurosis, beginning with some broad features of the psychoanalytic theory of personality.[8]

In psychoanalytic theory, it is assumed that psychological aspects of personality have a separate and important reality; that is, although all psychic processes do originate from the body, bodily processes alone cannot explain psychological variations among people and within the same person at different times. Bodily processes are not usually experienced directly; rather they are known through their psychological representation—that is, experientially. For example, in sexual arousal it is not the changes in heart rate, respiration rate, and activation of glandular and hormonal systems that are experienced but the psychological representation of these physical changes. We say, "I am in love with this person," not, "I now feel a change in my

---

[8] Students who wish to become more fully acquainted with psychoanalytic theory should consult the following references: O. Fenichel, *The Psychoanalytic Theory of Neuroses* (New York: W. W. Norton, 1945); R. Waelder, *Basic Theory of Psychoanalysis* (New York: International Universities Press, 1960). There are, of course, many other excellent books on this subject. Fenichel's book is very difficult to read, but it is quite complete. Students who are interested in becoming clinical psychologists should own a copy and should read it at various times in their training, because the ability to comprehend it grows with one's level of training. Waelder's book is an easier version of Fenichel's book; it is quick reading and speaks a "more modern language."

heart rate and hormonal balance." The language of psychology is that of experience. But psychological experience rests on physiological aspects of life.

Psychoanalysts consider sexuality and aggression to be the two most important psychological phenomena, closest to physiological aspects of the person. Sexuality and aggression are often referred to in psychoanalytic theory as the *basic drives*. They become differentiated with development and may become de-differentiated (fused again) with pathology even after they have become distinct. (Think of people who can experience sexual excitation only if there is physical cruelty.)

In terms of psychoanalytic theory, hunger and thirst are not good examples of basic-drive functioning. Sexuality and aggression are displaceable; hunger and thirst are not. Sexuality and aggression can be gratified in many ways other than directly; hunger and thirst eventually require actual food and drink for satisfaction. The facts that aggression and sexuality may be expressed in so many ways, that these drives infuse almost everything we do, and that early training has a profound effect on how they will serve or hinder the developing person render the basic drives a most important focus for students of personality development. (Note that in learning theories hunger and thirst are often referred to as "the drives." But learning theory uses very different concepts from psychoanalysis.)

In his early formulations, Freud was so impressed by the deleterious effect of withheld sexuality that he thought the experience of massive anxiety was a poisonous by-product of sexual repression. He regarded the repression of sexuality as the primary cause of neurosis. While we have come a long way from this formulation, it still has some value in that it underlines the powerful effect of child-raising practices and cultural values on personality formation. Recall that Freud worked with patients raised in the tradition of Victorian morality!

Anxiety still has a central place in the psychoanalytic theory of personality. Today it is viewed not as a toxic product of un-discharged sexuality but as a very painful psychological experience that may have many causes and a variety of effects.

What are some of the commonly known forms of anxiety? Freud thought that the earliest form of anxiety was experienced over the loss of the "love object"—that is, the caretaking person, the mother, the one who insures the infant's survival by feeding him, protecting him, and keeping him safe. Later, when survival is no longer so tenuous, anxiety over the loss of the love object may turn into anxiety over the possibility of loss of the love of an important person.

As the child grows older and develops desires that he fears might incur the anger of significant people, he may also experience anxiety over the possibility of being severely punished by them. For example, he might fear that his father will discover his secret—that he wants to have the mother all to himself and is rather glad when the father is away (perhaps he could be away all the time—perhaps he could just disappear and never come back!)—and that his father would then come and take away something very precious and personal! Who knows? Thoughts such as these can create a lot of anxiety when one is five years old.

As one gradually "incorporates" the values and standards of adults, one begins to develop a conscience. It is felt to be wrong to do certain things or to have certain thoughts, not because of fear of punishment by others, but because one knows that one will suffer: "If I do this, I know I will feel awful for the rest of the week"—this is anxiety over one's conscience. Later, in adolescence, one may become quite dismayed at the thought of "falling apart" or "going crazy" when the pressure of sexual and aggressive impulses is too great to handle and one feels overcome *by forces from within.* Clearly, there are many ways of talking about different kinds and degrees of anxiety.

We should not make the mistake of thinking of all anxiety

as neurotic or as naturally leading to neurosis. In deciding what is neurotic and what is normal anxiety, clinicians usually try to determine how justified the experience is. Suppose that you are visiting a friend and suddenly discover that a member of his family has measles. You then spend several days feeling anxious that you might have caught it. No one would say that this was neurotic anxiety; on the contrary, it could be said that your ego is performing its natural function of sending you messages of "signal anxiety," which under the circumstances would be a self-preserving experience. But if you were to worry over things that are not at all likely to happen to you and become incapacitated in everyday life because of such worries, then there might be reason to wonder, "Is it all justified and where will it lead you?"

Whatever its source, anxiety is a very painful experience and people will do almost anything not to experience it. The psychological maneuvers they engage in in order to avoid anxiety are called *defense mechanisms.* Generally, a person is not aware of his defense mechanisms. They are not used consciously. Healthy people have a great many defense mechanisms at their disposal and use them flexibly and without too much cost to adaptive, creative living. Very neurotic people (and who is not neurotic even to a slight degree?) use defense mechanisms at a great cost to happy and productive living. Moreover, the defenses they use do not function well; that is, they are still left prey to psychological discomforts and anxieties of many kinds.

Some children have a great deal of guilt over masturbating. They may have been told that it would make them sick, that if they were caught "doing that" their hands would be cut off, or worse. Yet they cannot help themselves. At night, when they are alone in bed, they become fearful, tense; they begin to play with themselves until they fall asleep. They may be aware of what they are doing and may be very anxious that someone will find out or that someone already knows. They feel they should not do it; they promise themselves that they will "never again" do it;

yet they continue to do this "dirty thing" rather regularly. (Note that in this example masturbation itself is a defense against night fears, which is often the case. But, we may assume, the children do not know they masturbate *because* they are afraid of the dark.)

After a while such children may have sufficient anxiety over their masturbation (and no one to talk to about it) that they develop a symptom—such as handwashing. It is as if someone were telling them, "You are dirty, your hands are dirty for touching yourself there. Go wash your hands!" They do not know why they always have to wash their hands. They just have to. For a while, after they have washed, they feel better—that is, relieved of their anxiety. But then the discomfort begins again and off they go to wash already clean and chapped and raw hands—in an unending cycle of sin and expiation. Psychologists would say that such children are trying to defend against anxiety in a very neurotic way, that the defense (handwashing) does not really help them, that the entire complex of night fears—masturbation-guilt-anxiety-handwashing—is maladaptive and rather a waste.

Anxiety and the defenses used against it may have a traumatic origin. Trauma is a difficult concept to define in a general way because what is a traumatic experience for one person may just be slightly trying for another. A trauma is an event that a person cannot handle at a particular time in his usual ways of meeting difficulties; thus trauma is always relative to "how it happened and to whom." Consider the case of a little girl who became gravely ill just when she was beginning to talk. She was rushed to the hospital and almost died there. She was kept in the hospital for several months, during which time she was subjected to painful medical procedures. She cried ceaselessly for her mother. Once recovered, and years later, she was still known as "timid" and "shy." She talked only when she had to. It was as if the whole matter of communication had become associated with her illness—"If you try to talk, to express yourself, to say things, to assert yourself and make your wishes known, the most horrible things are going to happen to you." Her illness, or rather its timing, induced in her a traumatic neurosis. Her defense against anxiety (not communicating) later interfered with her schoolwork and her ability to express her wishes. Note that the trauma in itself does not entirely account for the subsequent neurosis—it was a precipitant. The neurosis—being shy, withdrawn, nonassertive—was what she then "chose" as a way to avoid pain. This strategy did not save her pain, however, because she then had to suffer being seen as inadequate, stupid, and unpromising as a student. Ultimately she paid for anxiety reduction in the currency of loneliness.

No one really knows why a child who feels guilty over masturbation "chooses" handwashing as a neurotic defense, or why a traumatized little girl "chooses" withdrawal and shyness to ward off further danger. Other children with similar experiences turn out differently—they develop different neuroses or they are relatively healthy with only a few bad memories to mark the spot where anxiety used to be. This, then, is the real mystery of neurotic character formation: What determines the choice of defense?

The various types of neuroses listed under psychoneurotic disorders in the classification of the GAP report can be thought of as different from one another mainly in the *different constellations of defense mechanisms that characterize each.* These defense mechanisms in turn may be classified, or ordered. Most frequently, they are described as ranging in complexity. For example, avoidance is a relatively simple defense mechanism; isolation is more complex. Students of psychopathology spend a great deal of time trying to understand how these mechanisms "work" and trying to determine their possible correlates in the total personality. Let us consider a few examples of defense mechanisms.

Avoidance, as its name implies, means that the person turns away from, stays away from, will have nothing to do with, that which threatens to arouse anxiety. Avoidance occurs without awareness. It is not that the person decides, "From now on I will not look at . . . , talk with . . . , read about . . . ." Rather the person simply *avoids* threatening things, people, ideas. Note that in many instances the avoidance mechanism can be quite adaptive and economical. After all, no one can deal with everything head on or cope with every difficulty. Avoidance is neurotic when it is out of proportion and overgeneralized. It is neurotic, for example, in phobias, where not only originally anxiety-evoking matters are avoided but also those people, ideas, or things that are in some way associated with the source of anxiety. Thus a child who was once frightened by a dog in an elevator may now refuse to go into elevators, escalators, airplanes, or any other conveyance that rises. The avoidance may become so generalized that no one, least of all the child himself, knows what exactly he is afraid of.

Denial is a more complicated mechanism in which there is some commerce with the anxiety-arousing matter but then it is denied: "It is not that I am afraid of dentists, it is just that I do not like this particular doctor." Here reluctance is admitted, but not the dread of dentists in general.[9]

In middle class culture strong feelings, particularly angry feelings, are frequently denied awareness. It is not "nice" to be very angry. Children often feel deep anger, but they have been raised to deny their rage. When feelings are blocked from awareness, serious problems can arise. Excessive denial of feelings is found in many types of childhood psychopathology.

Repression is a defense mechanism in which an event, a feeling, or an idea is totally banished from awareness; none of it

[9] The statement about the dentist could, of course, be true. Its validity comes into doubt when, for example, a person has tried a succession of dentists, each time reaching the same conclusion: "Not dentists in general, just this one, and this one, and this one too. . . ."

leaves a mark on one's consciousness. Since repression plays a role to some degree in all defense mechanisms, it is sometimes considered the archetype of all defenses. Freud compared the pervasive use of repression to the military takeover of a revolutionary government. Instead of integrating the rebels into a new cabinet, the forces in power simply put them in jail. The implication of this analogy is that it takes effort to keep repressed material banished from awareness, and that what was once repressed may return suddenly and catch us unaware. Have you ever looked through an old trunk and discovered baby pictures of yourself, or an old poem you wrote as a child, or something else that you "know" was once part of you but that now no longer "feels" like part of you? It is a shocking and sometimes disturbing experience.

Isolation is a relatively complex defense mechanism. Sometimes we become anxious because a feeling belongs with another feeling, an idea with another idea, or a feeling with an idea to which we feel it "ought not" to belong. The mechanism of isolation is then put into effect to separate the two components; separately they can be tolerated. For example, at various times most children feel ambivalent about their parents. After all, parents give but also prohibit, they love but also punish, they help but also control. Young children cannot tolerate ambivalence; in a very real sense they are not ready for it. Children's stories abound in "fairy mothers" who are good, beautiful, bountiful, and sweet and "witch mothers" who are mean, frightening, and dangerous. In fantasies and in fairy tales children have a propensity to isolate the good from the bad, and only later do they learn to tolerate ambivalence and to accept the fact that most things, after all, are a mixture of both.

Children who have lost a parent early in life often bewilder those around them by a total absence of mourning. They may recall the *event* of the loss, but the *feelings of grief* are too dangerous to experience. The feelings are isolated from the event and may succumb to repression, or they may become attached to another event that is less devastating. Some clinicians believe that early loss, isolation, and repression of grief are responsible for the evolution of a life style of mild but chronic melancholy.

An entire volume could be written about the defense mechanisms found in children; in a very real sense clinical knowledge on this score is unsystematized. However, good beginnings have been made by those who publish their work in the *Psychoanalytic Study of the Child,* an annual publication of the International Universities Press. A more systematic discussion relevant to children may be found in Anna Freud's well-known classic, *The Ego and the Mechanisms of Defense,* the last edition (1960) being the best. These recommendations are mentioned here rather than in a footnote in order to underscore the importance of further reading on a complex topic that has been given only a brief introduction here.

A case of obsessive-compulsive neurosis in childhood

John was eleven years old, the only son of professional parents.[10] He was referred to a psychologist for evaluation because he was unable to learn in school and was about to fail his grade. His parents were aware of his school problems but were nevertheless shocked to find that matters in school had deteriorated to such an extent. They were willing to do anything to set things right. John was also somewhat worried about his difficulties in school, but he habitually promised his parents and himself that he would do better. The threat of failing was a surprise to him

[10] According to Principle 2.35-1 set forth in *Ethical Standards for Psychologists* (Washington, D.C.: American Psychological Association, 1953), essential details of this case have been altered to protect the patient's privacy.

too, and he received the news by making additional promises to work harder.

John was tall and spindly-looking, with thick glasses and good manners. He spoke with poise and a certain amount of disdain about psychology. Some of his friends had been taken to psychologists and as far as he could see they had gained little from it. However, he was willing to undergo some tests "just in case" he might find them "interesting."

John's developmental history was uneventful. He had had the usual childhood diseases. His eyesight was poor and he had been wearing glasses since the second grade. He had few friends and was known as a loner. He had not shown any interest in girls but was occasionally involved in sports. He said that his favorite activity was reading; in fact, he read quite well. Yet his mother reported that he often sat in front of an open book gazing out the window. Whenever she questioned him about what he was doing, he would claim that he was "thinking about things."

The Wechsler Intelligence Scale for Children showed John to have an IQ of 132, placing him in the "very superior" category for children his age—only slightly over 2 percent of children are this bright. Thus it was not possible to explain his failure in school in terms of deficient intelligence. On the contrary, his high score placed additional burdens on the psychologist: How can a child with "very superior" intelligence, who likes to read and is well-mannered and socialized, be on the brink of failing a grade in school?

We often hear the term *underachiever*. That there are children who "achieve below their potential" cannot be denied, but we should be cautious rather than cavalier in applying this term. Underachievement implies that when a child's intelligence far exceeds his achievement, the discrepancy is due to the child's failure to use his potential. But how is potential measured? Psychologists do not have a test for assessing intellectual potential. There are tests that give a quantitative index of how well a child can perform in relation to other children of his age; but how well he can perform depends in large measure upon how well he has been "learning," in a very broad sense of the word. School achievement is one measure of how well a child has learned; intelligence test results are another measure of learning. We may *infer* from a good test result that the child has strong capacities to learn, but we should always use caution in making the inference in reverse. Poor test performance can mean poor learning, for all the many reasons that children do not acquire knowledge. But to infer that children with low-measured intelligence *ipso facto* have a low capacity to learn is a dangerous conclusion.[11]

At any rate, in John's case the high IQ score explains nothing of his school failure and only complicates the clinical picture. Clearly, the psychologist must look elsewhere in his attempt to understand John's poor record in school.

John's attitude toward the psychologist remained casual and easy over five appointments. He continued to see his school problem as a transitory difficulty due to his having too many outside interests, and he believed the problem would surely clear up as soon as he "decided" to apply himself with more attention to the teacher's requirements. He thought his teacher was "all right" though at certain times too simplistic in her explanations and at other times unreasonably demanding of "boring and monotonous" work. He treated the psychologist in much the same tone, obliging in his responses and at times condescending. For example, when asked to speak more slowly so that his responses could be written down, he slowed to a dictation rate of speech, making it seem as though the psychologist were his secretary. All the while John was happy to oblige, finding this superior

[11] There has been much talk in education about the possible genetic meanings of low intellectual performance. Students with a special interest in this problem are encouraged to read M. Golden and W. Bridger, "A refutation of Jensen's position on intelligence, race, social class, and heredity," *Mental Hygiene*, 53 (1969), 648–53.

posture least dangerous to his self-esteem. He ended each testing hour by thanking the psychologist for his interest in him and saying that he had enjoyed himself, but always like someone liberated from an extremely boring social occasion.

Subsequently John was given many other tests, among them the Thematic Apperception Test developed by Henry A. Murray. In this test patients are shown a series of pictures and are encouraged to tell stories about them. The assumption is that TAT stories will reveal matters of personal concern—values, fears, aspirations, and preoccupations—that are not entirely conscious. The TAT is a very sensitive test, and as with all sensitive tests it will yield data that are "good" to the extent that there exists a good relationship between the patient and the psychologist and to the extent that the psychologist is skilled in interpreting the stories. A cautious or suspicious patient will give tight and guarded stories; he will not "let himself go" or "use his imagination," and even the richest and most revealing stories will not contribute to the diagnosis if the psychologist lacks the sensitivity or training necessary to "decode" their content.

Let us examine some of John's TAT stories and see how he reveals himself in them. The first picture in the test depicts a young boy contemplating a violin on a table before him. This is what came to John's mind when he looked at the picture:

> (After a laugh, and a pause.) This boy's father bought him a violin to take lessons so someday he could be a great violinist. He's looking at the fiddle wondering why he ever took it up. (Pause.) He does not like to practice. (Pause.) Of course, the outcome is that his father comes and makes him practice, which isn't pleasant. That's that. (The psychologist inquires whether the boy does become a violinist.) Yes, young David Oistrakh. His father figures he will support him in his old age. The boy begins to like practicing and does it four, five hours a day.

Compared with John's later stories this one is moderate in intensity. He is complying with the request to tell a story, but he does not yet "let himself go." However, we begin to get a glimpse of John as a boy for whom accomplishment may be an arduous affair. Practicing "isn't pleasant," and once success is achieved one has to assume responsibilities such as supporting one's parents. Note also that achievement is cast in less than modest terms—one does not just become a violinist, one "over-achieves" and becomes internationally famous. The question arises: What is the nature of John's relationship with his father? The story is unelaborated beyond the implication that conflicts in wishes between father and son are resolved by the son's compliance (overcompliance?) and a subsequent shift in dominance.

Note the formal qualities of the story. It begins with a tense laugh and a pause and ends with "That's that." The most significant part of the story emerges when the psychologist prods John to say more. He can and does put a stop to his ideas when he feels that he has said enough.

The next picture shows a woman looking into a room. The room contains a table with a lamp on it, and the door is ajar. Here is John's story:

> Hmmm, here is a picture I don't understand. (He is encouraged to think about it further.) This lady's young ones got into the room in which the lady will have a party. She previously told them to keep their hands off the clean white tablecloth. She did not tell them not to eat the daisy centerpiece. So she finds a dish full of beautiful green stalks and the kids licking their fingers. She put roses in place of the daisies—the kids couldn't eat that, too thorny. The kids were sent up to bed with no supper.

The image of the woman, the mother, is also lacking in warmth and responsiveness. A childish prank is countered by a somewhat muted retaliation (roses have thorns) and deprivation (no supper). Although anger is implied in the story in the acts of the mother, *feelings* of anger are absent. "The young ones," "kids licking their fingers"—such ways of referring to children are odd for one who is still a child himself. But perhaps he does not feel like a child and tries to represent himself as an adult might—slightly derisive of people who play pranks and who lick their fingers! Both stories so far have a joyless quality. Feelings of resentment are always implied but not openly stated.

The third picture shows a huddled figure with its back to the onlooker. A vaguely outlined object, easily perceived as a gun, is on the floor near the figure:

> Hmmm, good picture for a murder mystery. Should I go into a mystery? I don't think I should. This boy was whittling wood the wrong way. The knife slipped and gave him a gash. Went to a doctor . . . stitched it up . . . into a sling. In the picture he is sitting here, head in arm, gritting his teeth because it hurts so much, and he is looking at the knife and the unfinished whittling. After that he always whittled *away*. (Pause.) It takes long to build up a mystery. . . . It takes another five minutes to get the killing . . . then ten to give the (words lost) . . . scene. Takes an expert like Erle Stanley Gardner to do that.

Have you ever developed a photograph? The positive image emerges gradually as you move the negative around in the solution. So it is with making inferences from TAT stories. With this last story John is beginning to emerge as a person who is quite troubled about expressing aggression. Does he turn angry feelings inward (whittling the wrong way, gritting his teeth)? It was the boy's own fault that he got hurt and now there is no one to comfort him. He can and does resolve not to do it again. One learns in pain and in regret.

But what of the other story, the one he thought he *should not* tell? John decided to keep the murder mystery to himself. Did he really? In the theme of whittling, aspects of the murder story do appear (someone getting hurt, someone being sorry); the story he willed himself to tell cannot obliterate the one he wished to conceal. The unarticulated murder mystery returns at the end. Note that its reappearance is accompanied by thoughts of overachievement. Like David Oistrakh, Erle Stanley Gardner is the ultimate in his field. But such expertise requires the ability to carry out a "mission impossible," as the following story will confirm.

The next picture depicts in the foreground a young boy and next to him, propped against the wall, a gun; behind him is a hazily drawn picture of two men bending over a third who may be seen as dead or sick. One man has a pointed tool in his hand. This is John's story:

> Hmmm. (John whistles softly as he looks at the picture.) This is easy. This boy is the descendant of a great doctor who lived on an island and he is telling the story of how his father saved the life of a native. The doctor hadn't any good surgical equipment so he sharpened up his letter opener, boiled it. . . . While this—a storm started there were no shutters. The lanterns went out. He had a hard time taking out the appendix. But he managed to get it out. The native was all sewn up, then the storm quieted down. He feels a great sense of achievement. (John is asked to tell what would have happened if the operation had not turned out all right.) He would feel bad but not as bad as if the weather was good. The odds were against him. (What kind of man was the doctor?) This doc was the kind of man who is always willing to take a beating. Like in a native uprising. The natives did not want white doctor (pause) witchcraft (pause) so

there was an uprising. They came very near to killing him but he managed to convince them that he wasn't as bad as he thought he was.

Again John tells a story within a story: a doctor's son is describing something that happened to his father. It appears that the "TAT situation" (telling a story in response to some pictures) is not enough protection for John. He has to tell a story *within* that, to make the content twice removed. Again the theme of greatness appears—to Oistrakh and Erle Stanley Gardner John now adds a great doctor. What began on a passing note now reaches a crescendo: not only is great achievement difficult; it is also supremely costly. One might not only write about murder, one might in fact be murdered—unless, of course, one has the power to convince one's assailants that one is not "as bad as he thought he was." That is not a printing error. The "he" was John's unconscious feelings of guilt betraying him and emerging into the open. The fact that he did not bother to correct his slip of the tongue leads us to believe that he remained unaware of it even after he said it.

The effortfulness of the doctor's action is somewhat rewarded by a sense of achievement. But consider the price—no surgical tools, no shutter, a storm, no illumination, then an uprising. There is the threat to life, the accusation, and finally the self-justification. Hardly a joyful picture of a job well done and just rewards to the winner. To be that good one has to be willing always to take a beating. Is it worth it? The story implies that one really has no choice but to try to perform against all odds.

But should one lose, one may use rationalization: if the odds were against the doctor and he failed, he would not feel as bad as if the odds had been in his favor. Such thinking may well indicate that John's powers of rationalization are quite developed, as they well might be in view of the fact that he is bright and yet failing in school.

Note the absence of anger again. There is no reproach for the ingratitude of the natives or for the accusations of witchcraft, no resentment against the terrible circumstance; there is mainly the uphill struggle to come through somehow and to fulfill the terrible burden of the responsibility to help. One has to practice to become famous to satisfy the father. One has skill. One has to operate to save a life. One has to take a beating.

Let us see how these themes evolve through the last two stories. The next picture shows a youngish man turning away from a woman as if he wished to escape from her. The woman holds on to the man. In the background is the faint suggestion of the figure of another woman, small and lightly drawn in. Here is John's story:

Hey! These look familiar from the movies, especially that man. (Pause.) Well, during the war our hero has just received orders to go overseas. His lover is . . . holding him. . . . Last farewell, and he is looking toward his equipment, uniforms, guns, wondering what will become of him overseas. When overseas he was nearly captured by Japs, escaped from concentration camps. Then safely back to the U.S. camp. (Pause.) So just as he is getting into the U.S. camp a German volley brings him down. He is given the Purple . . . and sent to rest in the States. His lover is waiting. The outcome is that he gets back safely. (How?) He joined the Army first, to board the ship. (The lovers?) They met, fell in love, and were planning to get married a week after he left. She said she'll always be waiting for him. She told him the truth. After the war and discharge, he had nothing short of six medals. They got married. (What if he had not been so successful?) She probably would have left him alone, scolded him and left him. (And he?) He would go out and find another girl.

Note the slightly derisive tone, the mockery in the reference to "our hero," who has "nothing short of six medals." All the misfortunes befalling "our hero" are mentioned without much feeling. Emotions are also well hidden when John supposes that the love affair might go awry because of lack of achievement. The tale is told tersely and its sad content is kept at arm's length. The movie setting is an additional disguise. Children often use such a technique. "Long ago and far away in a distant land . . ." almost anything can happen without tragedy or horror touching us personally. Such mental constructions are called *distance devices* and they serve a defensive function. Recall that defenses are not pathological *per se*. But what John does with feelings in general has implications for understanding his total personality.

It is interesting to note that while John tells a love story along with the war story, he manages not to deal with *relationship*. At least not here. People promise to marry, they wait for each other, and if one of them does not "come through" people decide to marry someone else. It is all very simple. Events push people along much more than people move events.

The curious position of achievement in the story is hard to define. Heroic deeds do not protect people against misfortune. (In fact, John can conceive of a veritable bouquet of bad luck that accompanies heroism.) But lack of achievement can bring about the loss of all that is generally felt to be precious. The easy-come, easy-go quality of the story is its main significance.

With the presentation of the last TAT card John's tone changes. This is truly remarkable. The last picture depicts a boy sitting in the doorway of a log cabin:

> This child's mother and father . . . rather the mother
> had died three years before and his father isn't exactly
> nice to him. He is sitting out there feeling gloomy. The
> father punished him for doing nothing and he is sit-
> ting out on the steps wondering why his father is so

mean. The outcome is that his father marries a new lady. . . . This lady reforms his father. The lady is not fat, but taller and stronger than his father, and taught him a thing or two about how to treat children. She had some children of her own. The father got to be a real nice man. His half-brother and he had a lot of fun together. (What about the half-brother?) He had a much better life because *his* mother was kinder. He, the husband, he hadn't been divorced, someone actually shot him. . . . This man had . . . was a criminal and it is believed that the police snuck up behind him, giving him a bullet in the back. The little boy never knew his father . . . he was lucky. The half-brother had a much easier life. . . . The mother was kind . . . they all had their chores but they weren't punished when they made a mistake.

It is as if some kind of outside armor has fallen away. The lonesome little boy on the TAT card now elicits real feelings, deeply lodged longings, a kind of open wish for life to be different, for parents to be different, for having a brother to whom one can feel close. Reality is rearranged in thought and the wish becomes actuality: suddenly there is a reformed father, a new mother, a good brother, and an easier life.

Since the examining psychologist was a woman, we might wonder whether the new mother who "taught the father a thing or two about how to treat children" might not have been she, who after all was in the role of the helper to the boy in the actual clinical context of the testing.

With this last story John writes his own ticket—if there were another mother who could change the father into a more kindly man, and if the boy were not punished for minor omissions and commissions, life would become livable and even happy.

The remarkable aspect of this story is not only the content but the content *in the previous context* of achievement-oriented, driving, uncompromising themes. One stands in awe of the simple childish wish, which has to be masked by such laboriously invented complexities as his previous stories reveal. After all, what child has never had the wish and the fear that one of his parents might die? What child has never daydreamed that the particular set of parents he is "stuck" with will undergo some transformation, some magic change, after which everything will be all right? Children often have such fantasies. Since the parents they do have are so mean, so lacking in understanding, so unkind and severe, perhaps these are not really their *real* parents! No real parents could be this mean! Perhaps, who knows, one was a foundling, and somewhere there is a set of real and perfect parents. Or perhaps someone else's parents would make a better pair than the real ones; one could get adopted or run away. Perhaps one could die, and then at one's funeral *they* would wish they had been good and kind.

John's wish story originates from such sources. When life seems unlivable, the compromises unbearable, and the constraints totally unworkable, then at least on the level of wish-fulfilling fantasy life can be totally revised. Propelled by the wish, the process of thinking soars unhampered by guilt, which otherwise shackles the imagination. ("Shall I go into a mystery? I don't think I should.") People, events, and circumstances that stand in the way of the wish are simply eliminated (". . . the mother had died three years before") and seemingly unalterable realities are changed for the better ("The father got to be a real nice man"). On the level of wishing, everything becomes possible.

We might wonder: Why did John not tell this story earlier? Why did he tell it at all? Such questions are really inquiries about how his defenses function. The wish to have a totally different life with his parents seems not to be freely available to him. He cannot just think it out loud under any circumstances. Quite possibly, even in telling it he is not aware that he is articulating a wish of his own and not a wish of the boy in the picture.

This is, after all, a dangerous wish to tolerate on the level of conscious experience. That he told it at all is due both to the projective nature of the test, which allows him to reveal himself obliquely, and to his feeling safe, unjudged, and well liked in the testing relationship. Had the testing situation resembled in any way John's relationship with his father, whom he perceived as demanding and judgmental, he could not have produced many of these stories, and especially not the last one. He could not have relaxed his defenses.[12]

John's case was selected here as an illustration of neurosis in children because the nature of the clinical material makes it possible to show neurotic functioning in even a limited discussion. The student should realize, however, that psychological diagnoses require a good deal more material than was presented in this case. Usually, the psychologist works with the history of the child and of the parents and with several other types of test data. Often the inferences drawn from such information are much more complex than those made here. John's case just happens to be a good "teaching case" because even a portion of the clinical data allows us to demonstrate possible connections between his fantasy life and his failure in school.

[12] In evaluating the adequacy of diagnostic work with a child, the clinician must always be aware of the interpersonal and situational context of the testing. A clinical evaluation is a very delicate matter because it is really not the testing that generates data but the entire context of the relationship between the child and the adult. In this respect clinical evaluations are different from tests that some psychologists like to call "objective," meaning that the elusive and delicate aspects of the interpersonal relationship are kept out of the results. However, psychologists differ in what they consider "objective," just as they differ in what they consider "reliable." It is often argued that clinical tests are unreliable because they yield varying results depending on factors like the relationship between tester and patient. But it can also be argued that clinical tests above all should be sensitive tools responsive to feelings and attitudes. To the extent that a measuring device is sensitive, it might be variable and therefore "unreliable" by some standards.

Inferences are mental processes by which the psychologist attempts to "make sense" of clinical data so that he can connect his direct experience with the patient to a personality theory. There can really be no explanation without a theory. Even if the psychologist does not rely on a particular theory in his work, sooner or later he will have to bring some assumptions to bear on the data he collects. These assumptions may not be a theory in the sense that the psychologist does not weave them together in a systematic form, but they will of course affect his process of interpretation in some way. There can be no assumption-free explanation in clinical work. Clinicians simply differ in how explicitly they rely on one particular theory or another.

At any event, let us return to the case of John. The question before us is still: How can it be that a boy so bright is failing in school?

Of the two "basic drives," sexuality and aggression, the latter appears in many forms in John's thoughts. He attempts to deny feelings of anger. He decides to steer away from themes of murder. He turns anger against himself. He resolves, he tries, he promises. He hides resentment in humor and covers it with hints, implications, and rationalizations. He tries to keep themes of destruction at a distance. He adopts a derisive, superior tone toward people. Yet he seems to be tied to a preoccupation with anger. We infer from this that feelings of anger make him very uncomfortable, anxious, and perhaps guilty. He attempts to avoid this anxiety over anger by using a variety of defense mechanisms —denial, rationalization, and isolation. Since anger is nevertheless ever present in his productions, we infer that his defenses are not functioning well. He spends a great deal of energy trying to defend himself against anger but he is still uncomfortable about it.

The theme of achievement also recurs in John's stories. There is a preoccupation with heroic deeds, fantastic feats, impossible missions. Great undertakings in fantasy bring with them terrible burdens. Situations demanding great achievements are inevitable, as are the often untoward results of success. Even when success does not result in disaster, the rewards are often meager. When the rewards are rich by ordinary standards—"nothing short of six medals"—there is no joy in the victory; joy is minimized and made sour by sarcasm, derisiveness. Thus the struggle against angry feelings and the struggle for success have similar features: one tries and tries and tries again but one cannot really win! To put it another way: John finds himself in a psychological situation which requires him to fight on two fronts. He has to struggle against experiencing anger and he also has to struggle to attain extremely high standards of success. He cannot win these two fights at the same time.

In order to serve the goals of success one must have available large quantities of aggression. One must either use aggression in lavish and unmodified ways (by becoming a war hero) or use aggression in sublimated and creative ways (by becoming a famous writer or artist). At any event, one has to *use* aggression and not forever struggle against it and try to inhibit it.

Thus it is not hard to understand why John does so poorly in school. To the extent that one has troubles with aggression, one cannot learn. To learn requires the alteration of a passive and an aggressive attitude. It is necessary not only to *allow oneself to be taught* but also to go after, to acquire, to incorporate, *to make one's own, actively, aggressively.* Also as a learner it is necessary to work for intermediate goals. If on the first try only the heroic will do, one is doomed to failure. Famous violinists are not born. Born with talent, they are then made. By practicing, by being taught, and by rather strong feats of will power, they *gradually* attain success.

There is some evidence that John's problem with achievement is somehow related to his *perception of his father,* and that his troubles with aggression have to do with his *view of both parents* as ungiving, demanding, and essentially untrustworthy. Their

expectations are high, they do not give support or encourage-
ment, and they do not understand what children need from them.
How could a child please them? If he could please them with
smaller deeds, by being good and doing his chores, if he could
please them with less than heroic accomplishments, then perhaps
there could be some love, some warmth, a workable future in the
household.

The indictment of the parents is strong, open, explicit. We
must be careful, however, not to infer that for this reason all
John's problems are due to his parents' attitudes and the way
they are with him. Clinical data reveal the patient's perception of
significant others. Perceptions may be valid or they may be distorted. In John's case his perceptions of his parents were partially
correct; they were people with very high standards, but they had
much more warmth and sympathy for him and were capable of
much more understanding of him than he gave them credit for.

In what ways can we see in John the workings of *neurosis in
the obsessive-compulsive style?* With what certainty can we say
that if John is not treated he will grow up to become an obsessive-
compulsive adult? What *is* an obsessive-compulsive adult?

One recent and extremely readable description of the obsessive-compulsive style is that given by David Shapiro in *Neurotic
Styles* (1965). Shapiro discusses the many ways in which the
obsessive-compulsive has marshaled his resources to oppose his
instincts. He points out that the term *rigidity* has often been used
to refer to many aspects of the obsessive-compulsive's behavior—
his stiff social manner and his careful way of handling his body,
as well as the manner of his thinking. Shapiro gives many examples of the peculiar inattention of the obsessive-compulsive,
which makes people feel as though they cannot "get through" to
him. However, the inattention is apparent only because the
obsessive-compulsive does in fact pay attention, but he focuses
on selected aspects of his experience. Thus in relationships with
others he often seems distracted and distant.

The obsessive-compulsive also demonstrates rigidity in the intellectual sphere. He selects and pays particular attention to certain details of a problem, he is upset by seemingly insignificant inaccuracies, and he follows certain lines of reasoning doggedly even though they may have no utility. Another way of characterizing the intellectual functioning of the obsessive-compulsive is to describe the many ways in which flexibility or mobility of attention has become impossible for him. Shapiro puts it as follows:

> These people seem unable to allow their attention simply to wander or passively permit it to be captured. Thus, they rarely seem to get hunches, and they are rarely struck or surprised by anything. It is not that they do not look or listen, but they are looking or listening too hard for something else. (Shapiro, 1965, p. 28.)

The obsessive-compulsive adult is often intensely active at some kind of work. There is about his style of working a quality of "tense deliberateness, a sense of effort, and of trying" (p. 31). The person thus constantly feels taxed and burdened. Activities that for others are a source of play or joy are drawn into the obsessive-compulsive's effortful and deliberate manner of approaching any task. "The compulsive person tries just as effortfully to enjoy himself at play as he does to accomplish or produce at work" (p. 32). The pressure comes from within—pressure to achieve, to accomplish, to reach a goal; but the compulsive person experiences this pressure as coming from without. He feels pushed, compelled, obliged, to accomplish certain tasks; his most characteristic thought is, "I should."

Shapiro's description is most vivid regarding the problem of will and volition in the obsessive-compulsive neurotic:

In his psychology, self-direction is distorted from its normal meaning of volition or choice and deliberate, purposeful action to a self-conscious directing of his every action, to the exercise, as if by an overseer, of a continuous willful pressure and direction on himself and even, strange as it may appear, an effort to direct his own wants and emotions at will. . . . Every action, every direction is weighty, heavy with deliberateness, like an act of state. . . . Impulse, in this order of things, is not the initiator or the first stage of willful directedness and effort but its enemy. Thus, for these people, impulse or wish is only a temptation which can corrupt their determination, interrupt their work, interfere with what they feel they "should" want to be doing, or otherwise endanger their rigid directedness. They are, therefore, cut off from the sources that normally give willful effort its direction. . . . This style of activity and experience . . . also implies a kind of self-awareness, an awareness of the overseer sitting behind and issuing commands, directives, and reminders, that the obsessive-compulsive person is never without. (Shapiro, 1965, pp. 36–37.)

At this point we can begin to see many similarities between John's behavior and Shapiro's descriptions of the obsessive-compulsive adult. Recall John's struggle against impulse, the decision-making about what story should or should not be told, the effortful and joyless quality associated with achievement, and the tone of inevitability that permeated his stories. Recall also that he tended to interpret his school failure as a problem of the will; that is, he thought that once he decided to do his homework regularly his schoolwork would improve, thereby disregarding the many previous times he had made such resolutions without result.

Further similarities between John's present way of functioning and the obsessive-compulsive style emerge from Shapiro's discussion of the way in which the compulsive person functions according to some kind of perceived moral necessity. The obsessive-compulsive feels duty-bound to comply with various kinds of "authoritative opinion, rules, regulations, and conventions, and perhaps above all . . . a great assemblage of moral or quasi-moral principles" (p. 40). In this regard, recall the choicelessness of John's TAT characters, the manner in which they fit in with role expectations held out to them by others, the way in which they play out their destiny as though following a script. This feature of his fantasies reaches a crescendo in the doctor story, in which moral necessity and professional role combine to dictate the doctor's behavior. More genuine, affectively determined commitment, such as love for his patient, is not the major influence on the doctor's behavior. Rather he finds himself in circumstances that allow him little choice but to operate.

With respect to the sense of reality, to that which is felt to be real, and the manner in which one relates to selected aspects of reality, Shapiro says the following about the obsessive-compulsive style:

> When one observes obsessive-compulsive people closely or examines their ideas or statements, it becomes clear that such a question as "Does it feel true?" or "Is it really so?" is typically answered neither one way nor the other, but is avoided. Even regarding matters about which he entertains no active doubt, the obsessive-compulsive person will often seem surprised by such a question and virtually dismiss it as irrelevant to his interest. He will not say, "It is true," but will say something like, "It must be" or "It fits." . . . One compulsive patient, for example, said of the girl he plans to marry, "I must be in love with her—she has all the qualities I want in a wife." . . . A sense of conviction about the world—a sense of truth, in other

words—involves a breadth of attention, an interest in
and sensitivity to the shadings and proportions of
things, and a capacity for direct response to them for
which the obsessive-compulsive person is not geared.
(Shapiro, 1965, pp. 50–51.)

All this brings us to the captive, repressed nature of John's
feelings. In terms of psychoanalytic personality theory, when certain kinds of affective experiences are dangerous, not only are the
dangerous affects blocked out of awareness but other feelings as
well. Although John's main problem with feelings seems to be his
difficulty in accepting anger and in dealing with it, he treats
other feelings—such as affection, love, and attachment—in a similar repressive way. To the extent that feelings are not available
to experience, life is desiccated of emotional realities and the
conscious experience is often one of boredom. John's sense of
boredom emerges not only from direct interview material not referred to here but also from his massive efforts to appear uncon-
cerned, matter-of-fact, and cavalier. Often when people present
themselves as offhand, uncaring, uninvolved, and indifferent, one
may infer that this is not just a pose or a conscious effort at de-
ception but that the sources of this behavior reside in a familiar
internal state of chronic boredom.

From this point of view—that is, considering repression of
feeling as a major impediment in John—the last story, though
sad, contains the best prognostic sign. In it John is able to show
open connection with feelings, wishes, yearnings, and disappointment, and is even able to describe pleasure.

The connection between the beginning signs of an obsessive-
compulsive neurosis in a very bright boy and the fact of school
failure is not difficult to draw. We can assume that John must
expend vast quantities of effort to maintain repression over aggression and that his intellectual work suffers for at least two
reasons in this regard: (1) when aggression is repressed it is not

available to be enlisted in the effort to learn; (2) the very attempt at repression requires effort that might otherwise serve curiosity and discovery.

Admittedly, this explanation of how John functions leaves out several important considerations. For example, because his case was used only for illustrative purposes we have not considered the manner in which his actual, real-life relationship with people impedes his functioning in school. But perhaps it will be clear from this limited amount of material that John has not yet found a comfortable way to relate to his parents and possibly to other adults. On one level, he wishes to be close, to be accepted, and to be loved. On another, he sees people as demanding and extracting of superhuman performance yet at the same time as weak, dependent themselves, and retaliatory toward those who express impulse. Somewhere between the reality of John's wishes and the reality of his perception lies a region in which he could engage in a healthy give-and-take, in a live and lively commerce with others in which people are more realistically perceived and experienced than either his wishes or his present perceptions will allow.

For all these reasons, psychotherapy was recommended for John with the primary aim of helping him to make friends with his own anger and of teaching him how to relate in a close, intimate relationship. It was hoped that a long-term, corrective emotional experience with a skilled therapist would help him to relinquish his present strategy of inhibition and overstriving and thus enable him to make better use of himself as a learner. One major reason for prescribing psychotherapy was not only to help him over his poor school performance but also to forestall an eventual obsessive-compulsive adjustment that, to be sure, might have had no adverse social consequences but that would have put a very low ceiling on his potential enjoyment of life.

CHAPTER THREE

Therapeutic Aspects

Variety of approaches to child therapy

There are many forms of psychotherapy for children. The purpose of this chapter is to present the student with a general view of the therapeutic aspects of clinical work with children. Because child therapy is as yet an unsystematized area of clinical functioning, it is difficult and indeed undesirable to impose upon this discussion a degree of cohesion that the field itself does not yet possess. As in the previous discussion of diagnostic work with children, we will examine the shape of the area of child therapy in broad outlines and then concentrate on selected forms of therapy.

Each approach to child therapy is based on certain assumptions concerning the causes of mental illness in children and the possibilities of altering the course of development gone awry.

However, these assumptions are not always explicit, and it is often difficult to see the connection between a particular method and the theory of developmental psychopathology underlying it. To be sure, every form of child therapy expresses beliefs and attitudes about mental illness and health, about the role of parents in the child's illness, and about the importance of the environment in causing or altering pathological development. Also, and more broadly stated, each form of psychotherapy expresses certain convictions about human nature and the value, importance, and violability or inviolability of personal choices.

Such matters find expression in the explicit or implicit goals of child therapy—as, for example, the preference for long-term work with "character problems" over short-term therapy with overt behavioral symptoms. Some therapeutic goals are mutually exclusive. For example, a therapist clearly cannot pay homage to the respective values of character alteration and symptom inhibition at the same time. Other goals of child therapy are not mutually exclusive. Thus a therapist may believe in the importance of individual work with children and may also be quite convinced that the family has to help in revising deleterious environmental circumstances; these two convictions may lead the therapist to combine individual with family therapy. The fact that certain goals can and do coexist and that various methods may be combined, together with the fact that methods as well as goals are often implicitly held rather than clearly spelled out convictions, lend the area of child therapy a multidimensional and richly textured quality.

The varieties of belief in child therapy can perhaps best be viewed in terms of the different schools of thought and individuals who, either singly or in combination, have been important influences on the psychotherapy of children. For example, Carl Rogers (1951) has had a considerable and palpable effect upon the field of child therapy, particularly through the work of Virginia Axline (1947). Her formulations of *nondirective therapy* rest on the belief that children come to deal with their anxieties as they grow more and more comfortable in a permissive and non-intrusive two-person relationship. Thus the aim of therapy is to create an atmosphere in which the child feels secure and unthreatened, on the assumption that with anxiety at a low ebb the child will explore his problems on his own terms and in his own time.

Recent developments in the application of conditioning techniques to the field of therapy have produced a new approach, called *behavior therapy* or *conditioning therapy*. The primary aim of this form of therapy is to inhibit or alter the objectionable symptoms from which the child suffers. (Browning and Stover, 1971.) While the field of behavior therapy is quite new, it has gained rapid popularity because it appears to bridge the gap between the preoccupation with illness in clinical psychology and the behavioristic orientation of developmental psychology. The name of this approach can be misleading, however, since every kind of therapy is behavior therapy in one sense or another. Therapies differ in how important they consider the mere alteration of behavior to be.

The formulations of *psychoanalytic theory* have long exerted an important influence on the field of child therapy both through the psychoanalysis of children and through less intensive, dynamically oriented individual therapy. The goal of psychoanalysis is long-range character revision and reorientation of defenses through the tools afforded by an intensive long-term relationship with the patient.

Given the three distinct kinds of convictions about child therapy represented by the nondirective, behavioral, and psychoanalytically oriented approaches, it should be clear that controversies about the adequacy of one technique over another can run along many channels and bring to the fore disagreements about broad values. There are many practical arguments and questions as well. For example, if psychoanalytic formulations are indeed adequate, why do many children treated by analytic methods for long periods of time fail to improve? Are the techniques of nondirective therapy really so different from other techniques? Is there not a great overlap between the permissive attitude of the nondirective therapist and the atmosphere created in the consulting room of a psychoanalytically oriented therapist, even though the latter will ask questions and offer interpretations to the patient and the former will not? Finally, is behavior therapy really so new? We have known for a long time that behavior can be altered rapidly by drastic methods. It is true that enuresis, tics, and other symptoms can be inhibited through the methods of conditioning, but why call symptom inhibition therapy? Of course it is good to be free of symptoms, but how do we know that these symptoms will not reappear in other, more complex forms at a later time in the child's life?

In the absence of definitive studies, or even of empirical work with minimal qualifications as well-controlled research, such questions and arguments remain in the realm of competing systems of belief. Lately there has even been disagreement about who is really the patient when a child is mentally ill. If we believe that noxious family relationships can cause mental illness in children, why not treat the family along with the child, or the family in the total context of its daily environment? Such arguments have given rise to the field of *family therapy*, one of the newest approaches.

Other disagreements involve environmental factors. If bad neighborhood conditions and inadequate housing, together with poverty, can account for at least a portion of mental illness in children, what good does it do to remove the child from this setting, treat him in a residential environment, and then upon his improvement return him to his former world? Some clinicians maintain that mentally ill children are not in a position to cope with the environment that made them ill until they are at least partially cured; others believe that if the child is not taught to stay in his own world, the cure is really just a way of socializing him in terms of more livable environmental conditions. A deprived child treated in a poverty-free setting might deteriorate upon his return home. This belief has given rise to the techniques of *educationally oriented residential treatment,* which provides the child with continuous contact with the home and the family.

The field is new. Much is not known. Methods are often tentative explorations into vaguely defined terrain. Goals of therapy are posed against conflicting conceptualizations about the evolution of psychopathology. Yet the possibilities of helping emotionally distressed children to overcome various kinds of developmental impasses are challenging enough to attract many young people to the field of child therapy.

Therapists may be trained in the medical profession as psychiatrists or psychoanalysts; or they may be trained in psychology, with a specialty in clinical child psychology. Social workers may also become child therapists with postgraduate training. Increasingly, child therapists are emerging from the ranks of educators and child care workers. Graduate as well as undergraduate students are showing increased interest in helping children. Often, either as tutors or as therapists in training, they achieve remarkable results.

Child therapists may function in private practice, hospitals, schools, or other educational institutions, or in connection with juvenile courts. There is a shortage of personnel in child therapy for all age groups, but nowhere is the lack of therapists as evident as with children in the elementary grades and below. This is because most therapists are trained to deal with adult patients and few ever "move over" to work with young children, although they often treat adolescents, whom they regard as "young adults."

There is little formal knowledge or research evidence about the personal qualities that enable some adults to relate to children with emotional problems while others, in spite of good intentions, fail to "connect" with youngsters. It is easier to intuitively select from a group of young people those who will work well with children than to explain exactly what it is that sets them aside from others not likely to succeed.

It is not enough to like children. One must also be able to accept primitive behavior without becoming either threatened or overly fascinated by it. It is necessary to understand play, and to use it intuitively. One must be able and willing to remember the frustration and unhappiness of one's childhood without perceiving every patient as necessarily suffering from the same problems. While it is important to identify with the child's difficulties in his family, one must not overidentify to the point of hating all parents or being unable to understand their life problems as adults. It is good to be open and free in emotional expression, but it is also essential to know when children need limits on their behavior. One must feel that the patient is very important as a person, but one cannot give so much of oneself that the child can never really do enough in return. The affections of the child should not be courted, yet it is equally important never to inadvertently reject a child's expressions of love. One must care deeply about one's patients, and when they are no longer in need of therapy one must also be able to let them go.

In this chapter attention will be given to two forms of individual therapy (psychoanalysis and intensive individual therapy) and to family therapy and educationally oriented residential treatment. Material related to forms of therapy not discussed here is cited in the reading list at the end of this book.

The following discussion should be viewed in the larger context of six major approaches to the psychotherapy of children:

1. Individual psychotherapy
   a. psychoanalysis
   b. intensive psychotherapy
   c. therapeutic tutoring

d. behavior therapy
2. Group therapy
3. Family therapy
4. Day hospital treatment
5. Residential treatment (medical orientation)
6. Residential treatment (educational orientation)

The psychoanalysis of children

Compared with other forms of therapy for children, psycho-analysis is relatively uncommon because it is very costly and be-cause there are very few analysts who work with young children. Psychoanalysis is considered most effective with youngsters who suffer from neurotic disturbances. Lately attempts have been made to adapt its techniques to treating children whose illnesses are more severe.

Children in analysis may see their therapists four or five times a week for several years. This creates an intense relationship, a degree of attachment between patient and therapist without which analysis is impossible. The parents are not part of this intense relationship, but it is necessary that they accept it and sanction it in order for treatment to proceed. The parents may have occasional talks with the child's analyst, or they may be seen by another clinician on a regular basis, even if they are not in treatment themselves. Since children in analysis often appear to become more disturbed before they get better, it is important that parents be given help in understanding the changes in the child.

There are many reasons why child analysis was first designed for, and is still primarily used with, children who have neurotic problems. The child must be able to use the explanations (inter-pretations) of the analyst; thus he has to be fairly bright and verbally oriented. Since psychoanalytic interpretations as well as the intense relationship with the analyst often create anxiety, the child must be capable of tolerating the discomfort. John, whose case was discussed in the previous chapter, was an excellent candidate for child analysis, because he was verbal and bright and functioned in a reality-oriented way in everyday life. That is, he would have brought enough strengths to treatment to make such an intense and "deep" method possible. Children with a tenuous hold on reality and weak controls over their impulses are generally not considered good candidates for child analysis, though this belief is changing, as we will see below.

The first case of child analysis on record is that of Little Hans. While the methods and theory of child analysis have undergone many changes since Sigmund Freud first published the case in 1909, the treatment of this little boy, who suffered from paralyzing phobias, remains a classic.

The case of Little Hans was unique in many respects. Although Freud directed the course of the analysis, the treatment was actually carried out by the father, a physician himself. He took careful notes about Little Hans's dreams, the questions the child asked, outside events, and conversations between himself and the boy. These notes were shared with Freud, who helped to unravel the mystery of Little Hans's intense fear of horses and other large animals, which first developed around the age of five. The published report gave a detailed account of dialogues between father and son, with commentaries by Freud.

The case of Little Hans was also unusual in that there was a "follow-up." As a young man, Hans came to see Freud and discussed his treatment with him. Freud was able to ascertain that the young man was completely free of his earlier symptoms, that he did not recall his treatment, and that he had sought out his former therapist only when he thought he recognized himself in the published version of the case! Students who are interested in working with children could hardly spend their time in a better way than in thoughtful reading of this unusual case. A few excerpts must suffice here.[1]

The following dialogue between Little Hans and his father illustrates the use of interpretation in one instance. Hans and his father had just been to a zoo, where Hans fearfully avoided visiting large animals, like giraffes and elephants. Prior to his disturbance, he had been quite fond of large animals, but this time he wished to see only small ones. The father reported the following exchange:

> I therefore said to him: "Do you know why you are afraid of big animals? Big animals have big widdlers, and you're really afraid of big widdlers."
> Hans: "But I've never seen the big animals' widdlers yet."
> I: "But you *have* seen a horse's and a horse is a big animal."
> Hans: "Oh, a horse's often. Once at Gmunden [summer place] when the cart was standing at the door, and once in front of the Head Customs House."
> I: "When you were small, you most likely went into a stable at Gmunden. . . ."
> Hans (interrupting): "Yes, I went into the stable every day at Gmunden when the horses had come home."
> I: "And you were most likely frightened when you saw the horse's big widdler one time. But there's no need for you to be frightened of it. Big animals have big widdlers, and little animals have little widdlers."
> Hans: "And everyone has a widdler. And my widdler will get bigger as I get bigger, because it does grow on me." (S. Freud, 1959, pp. 176–77.)

[1] S. Freud, "Analysis of a phobia in a five-year-old boy," in *Collected Papers,* vol. 3, Ernest Jones, ed., Alix and James Strachey, trans. (New York: Basic Books, 1959).

Sometime later the father reported a new way in which Hans was trying to deal with his fear of horses:

> "For some time Hans has been playing horses in the room; he trots about, falls down, kicks about with his feet and neighs. Once he tied a small bag on like a nose-bag." (S. Freud, 1959, p. 194.)

After several months and with much help from Freud, who saw the child on only a few occasions, it became clear that Little Hans's fear of large animals was a form of castration anxiety, and that his phobia included anxiety about the birth of babies as well as about sexual behavior among adults. Hans's recovery was marked by a fantasy that he told his father:

> ". . . The plumber came; and first he took away my behind with a pair of pincers, and then gave me another, and then the same with my widdler. He said: 'Let me see your behind!' and I had to turn around, and he took it away; and then he said: 'Let me see your widdler!' "

Hans's father grasped the nature of this wish fantasy and did not hesitate a moment as to its interpretation:

> I: "He gave you a *bigger* widdler and a *bigger* behind."
> Hans: "Yes."
> I: "Like Daddy's; because you'd like to be Daddy."
> Hans: "Yes, and I'd like to have a moustache like yours and hairs like yours. . . ." (S. Freud, 1959, p. 240.)

It would be a mistake to think that the spectacular case of Little Hans succeeded in initiating child analysis as a legitimate or popular subspecialty of psychoanalysis. While analytic theory always relied heavily on formulations concerning the role of childhood experiences in the origin of neurosis, concerted interest in treating children did not emerge among analysts until 1926. At that time there was a general widening in the scope of psychoanalytic theory, with new interests in delinquents, criminals, and psychotics; concern over the treatment of children was among the fresh topics under discussion. The newly formed Vienna Psychoanalytic Institute invited Anna Freud to deliver four lectures on the treatment of children under the title "Introduction to the Technique of the Analysis of Children." Many analysts attended the lectures, as well as students from America. Among them were men and women who later made major contributions to the field and whose names should be well known to readers of this book: Erik H. Erikson, Marianne Kris, Margaret Mahler, Marian Putnam, and Margaret Ribble.

Early in the development of child analysis attention was focused on the education of teachers, in an attempt to make psychoanalytic formulations relevant to practical applications with normal children. The Vienna Course for Educators had an effect on many American developments, such as the establishment of the Nursery School at the James Putnam Clinic in Boston, the Child Study Center at Yale University in New Haven, the Child Development Center in New York, and numerous other training and research facilities. However, it was not until after World War II that the separate training of child analysts actually began, at the Hampstead Clinic in England.[2]

---

[2] These historical developments were summarized by Anna Freud in a brief speech at the first meeting of the American Association for Child Psychoanalysis in Topeka, Kansas, in April 1966. They were published later that year. See A. Freud, "A short history of child analysis," in *The Psychoanalytic Study of the Child,* vol. 21 (New York: International Universities Press, 1966), pp. 7–14.

No adequate discussion of analytic therapy with children can be made without at least a brief look at the work of Anna Freud. Her pioneering contributions to the theory of treatment, diagnosis, education, and training are without parallel, and her major works continue to be a solid source of reading in the education of psychoanalysts.[3] These writings help us to gain a picture of the difference between child analysis as a treatment technique and the developmental theory on which it rests, and they make modest claims for the utility of the technique as compared with the broad-ranging applications of the theory.

Regarding the technique of treatment, Anna Freud is careful to point out that there are fundamental differences as well as similarities between the treatment of children and adults. For example, because the child is not a free agent and is still dependent on his parents, the analyst must have the parents' cooperation, and the child must know that his parents sanction his intense attachment to the analyst:

> . . . The analysis of children . . . must for the present be confined to the children of analysts, or of people who have been analysed or regard analysis with a certain confidence and respect. . . . Where a child's analysis cannot be organically grafted onto the rest of his life, but is intruded like a disturbing foreign body into its other relationships, more conflicts for the child may be created than can be resolved by the treatment. (A. Freud, 1946, p. 50.)

---

[3] Among Anna Freud's major works are *Psychoanalytical Treatment of Children* (London: Imago, 1946), containing the four famous lectures delivered in 1926; *The Ego and the Mechanisms of Defense* (New York: International Universities Press, 1960), now in its twelfth printing; and the most recent work, *Normality and Pathology of Childhood* (New York: International Universities Press, 1965), which contains several original formulations concerning the difference between normal developmental deviations and psychopathology.

In addition, because the child's personality is still in its formative stages and his controls over his impulses are relatively weak, the analyst cannot be solely devoted to "liberating" the impulses. The analysis should not become "the child's charter for all the ill conduct prohibited by society" (p. 49). The analyst must always be careful not to make the child's "real" life impossible through too much permissiveness, but at the same time he must encourage the emergence of impulses from behind the neurotic defenses erected against them. This double responsibility to "allow and forbid" is a delicate matter, a problem particularly attendant on the analysis of children.

The chief difference between child and adult analysis resides in the relative ease of the former over the latter:

> We can bring about quite other modifications of character in the child than in the adult. The child, who under the influence of its neurosis has started out on the path of an abnormal character-development, need only retrace its steps a short distance in order to find the road which is normal and suited to its nature. It has not like an adult built up its whole life, chosen its calling, made friends, fallen in love, chosen its ideals, all on the basis of its neurotic tendencies. In the "character analysis" of an adult we must actually shatter his whole life, and achieve the impossible, that is, undo things already done, and not only make ignored mental processes conscious but abolish them altogether—if we wish for real success. Here the analysis of children has an infinite advantage. (A. Freud, 1946, p. 50.)

The major disadvantage of child analysis is that children generally do not free-associate. However, they do play, and from their play one can often infer the repressed mental content, wish or fear. Since children dream and can report their dreams to the analyst, the technique of dream interpretation can be used with them. As Anna Freud often notes, children derive great pleasure from learning the significance of their dreams.

Recent attempts to extend the technique of child analysis to children with psychotic and borderline psychotic conditions[4] show that it is possible to modify the classical analytic technique of interpretation and verbal communication between child and therapist, and that such modifications "work" in the sense that they facilitate the development of a "therapeutic alliance" even with children who have shown deep disturbance in their willingness and ability to relate to people. These new applications of psychoanalysis promise not only to broaden the range of analytic techniques but also to provide new insights about the nature of borderline and psychotic conditions in children.

The contributions of Rudolf Ekstein are outstanding in clarifying dilemmas of therapeutic technique and personality theory. His recent volume, *Children of Time, Space, Action, and Impulse* (1966), brings together several important papers on the subject of borderline and psychotic children and offers ample illustration of what is meant by the modification of psychoanalytic technique.

For example, Ekstein describes how verbal communication must often be bypassed for the sake of symbolic action. He cites one case involving a six-year-old borderline psychotic boy. During a treatment hour the child invited the therapist to play "eat-

---

[4] As the name implies, borderline children are not as sick as psychotic youngsters. Their alienation from reality is not complete; they struggle to maintain themselves in the face of pathology. Because psychotic and neurotic aspects of their personality coexist and alternate—sometimes several times during the day and even during the therapy hour—their treatment offers particular challenges and problems. For an elaboration of the diagnostic aspects of working with borderline children see M. Engel, "On the psychological testing of borderline children," *AMA Archives of General Psychiatry*, 8 (1963), 426–34.

ing lunch together." At one point during the make-believe the child climbed on the table, slipped, and fell off. It all happened very suddenly and the therapist was not able to catch him before he hurt himself. After the child picked himself up off the floor and the therapist expressed concern and sympathy about his bleeding lip, the child turned angrily to the therapist and declared that he, the therapist, could no longer have any lunch. No amount of explanation about how it could not have been helped, how he could not have been caught, sufficed. The child acted as though the therapist had inflicted the injury upon him. Finally, the boy handed the therapist an empty Coke bottle and instructed him to eat it, as if to say, "Now that my lips bleed, and it was your fault, I will make your lips bleed too." The therapist played out eating the empty bottle. He reported:

> . . . I started to cry like the child had been crying. I cried out aloud, "My tooth, my tooth, nobody cares about me, nobody wants to catch me. Nobody cares, I'm all alone, I'm all alone." Jack regarded me with great animation and encouraged me to go on. "Pretend you got another tooth knocked out, then another." I did so and continued to lose lots and lots of teeth. Finally the child said relentingly, "You may have some chocolate milk." I thanked him profusely for the imaginary chocolate milk which he gave to me, and as I was drinking, Jack said suddenly, "Will you catch me if I fall?" Without any more notice, he jumped up on the play table with great rapidity, and threw himself headlong into space. Again he made no move to protect himself against the impact of the fall. By what seemed to be a miracle, this time I caught the child and I twirled him around several times saying that I had caught a lovely little boy and I was so glad that he had let me catch him. Jack laughed happily. (Ekstein, 1966, p. 154.)

Borderline psychotic children often communicate their worries, conflicts, fears, and secret thoughts very indirectly. The disguise of play is often not enough for them, and the make-believe thoughts and actions become quite "real." This poses new problems for technique, since the analyst obviously does not wish to credit the reality of such fantasies and at the same time does not want to risk rejecting the child by challenging the reality of his thoughts. Ekstein examines such newly discovered dilemmas in the psychoanalytic treatment of children and demonstrates novel ways of dealing with them in several cases described by himself and his associates. The most famous of these cases is that of the Space Child, which, as the name implies, concerns the long-term treatment of a boy whose entire fantasy life was invested in outer space fantasies.[5]

When first taken on in treatment, the Space Child was eleven years old. He had suffered from severe asthmatic attacks since the age of twenty-one months. He could not play. He was not able to get along with other children. His parents could no longer cope with his rebellious behavior. He could not be reassured that his fears of impending disasters would not materialize. In his fantasies he imagined himself as a five-star general who commanded countless spaceships and was out to destroy the world.

The detailed accounts of the treatment of the Space Child culminate in a report of follow-up contacts with him when he was in his twenties. As a young man he was still shy and somewhat tense; however, he was working for his Ph.D. in physics, was married, and had a teaching job. He had traveled in Europe and had handled his investment from an inheritance with success.

---

[5] Papers concerning the Space Child may be found in R. Ekstein, *Children of Time, Space, Action, and Impulse* (New York: Appleton-Century-Crofts, 1966), and should be read as "tomorrow's classics" by all those with a serious interest in the psychopathology of childhood.

Intensive psychotherapy

As we have seen, child analysis can be defined in terms of certain attributes of its method, such as high frequency of contact, interpretive comments by the therapist about the child's unconscious wishes, and the analyst's training. Intensive psychotherapy with children cannot be defined in this manner. It may be combined with other forms of therapy, may be given in an outpatient or a hospital setting, and may be directed toward many goals, ranging from attempting to redirect the child's evolving character structure to helping him to adjust more easily to a new life situation. Intensive therapy with children is best viewed as combining some of the methods and concepts of child analysis with some of the concepts and approaches of less intensive approaches to the therapy of children, often called "counseling." Counseling, intensive therapy, and child analysis can generally be regarded as existing on a *continuum of intensity,* marked by increasingly ambitious goals, more frequent contact, and increasing reliance on dynamic concepts in understanding the patient.

Since intensive therapy is currently the most common form of treatment, let us consider some of the events that might lead a child to it. His parents may be having marital problems and may initiate family therapy; the child may then be sent to individual treatment by the family therapist out of concern that his secret feelings about his parents' quarrels are not being properly explored in family therapy. Or a child may be sent to a psychoanalyst for intensive therapy by a pediatrician who has become concerned about the child's behavior. An adolescent might turn to his school counselor for advice about which college to choose. The counselor might be sensitive to underlying problems that stand in the way of making a sound career choice and might suggest psychotherapy to the young person instead of counseling.

The following discussion considers several aspects of child

therapy that often receive attention among clinicians and that invariably become foci in the supervision of student therapists. These aspects include the initial phase of child therapy, levels of communication in treatment of children, the importance of limits, and problems of termination. The aim of this discussion is to impart to the student an overview of this area of clinical functioning; no attempt has been made to give a definitive formulation.[6]

Initial phase—the "open" diagnosis

The psychological diagnosis of a child patient helps to rule out certain forms of treatment and to suggest others. A child diagnosed as schizophrenic is more likely to be in residential treatment than a child diagnosed as neurotic. A bright neurotic child is more likely to be in psychoanalysis than one with less intellectual skill. Of course, factors such as the economic circumstances of the family also play a part in determining what form of treatment is chosen. But aside from such practical considerations, the diagnosis points the way to particular kinds of treatment.

It is important to note, however, that what is known about the child at the conclusion of the diagnostic study can *chart the*

---

[6] The literature of clinical psychology does not offer a definitive text on child therapy, but there are a number of edited volumes containing good papers on selected aspects of child therapy. The student will find M. Haworth, *Child Psychotherapy* (New York: Basic Books, 1964), as well as M. M. Hammer and A. M. Kaplan, *The Practice of Psychotherapy with Children* (Homewood, Ill.: Dorsey Press, 1967), of interest. These two volumes contain papers by well over fifty specialists on such topics as the treatment of psychosomatic disturbances, phobias, compulsions, and hysterical conditions. The use of play materials and of various play techniques, problems of termination, and nonverbal communication are some of the many topics therapists write about.

course of treatment only to a limited extent. In the first two or three months of therapy children reveal more and more of themselves. The original diagnosis may undergo revision or it may be elaborated by the therapist to a fine level of understanding. For this reason, the initial diagnosis has to stand in a dynamic relationship to the first few weeks or months of treatment, during which time the therapist's own psychological posture toward the patient is best left flexible and open to new questions and new understandings.

Consider the case of a nine-year-old boy who was sent to intensive therapy with the diagnosis of school phobia. As the boy began to feel comfortable with his therapist and was encouraged to talk about his fears and his worries, he revealed that he was almost always mildly apprehensive when he was not at home. The child was fearful of going to school, but he was also "nervous" about being in crowds, being on the bus, and playing outdoors. The initial diagnostic study eliminated a number of possible explanations for the boy's poor performance in school: he did not have brain damage; he was not retarded or disturbed to psychotic proportions. But the positive initial diagnosis of school phobia appeared to be an understatement of the extent of the child's fearfulness. The initial diagnosis was not really a misdiagnosis; it was an underdiagnosis, if you will. It served to direct the therapist's attention very quickly to the possibility that where there is one phobia there are sometimes more.

After the initial phase of treatment, the therapist concluded that his main job was to discover the cause or causes of all the child's fears and apprehensions. The aim of therapy broadened. The initial goal had been to find out why the child was afraid of school in order to help him overcome his school phobia; under the revised diagnosis of a generalized phobic state, new understandings were sought about the boy's feelings regarding his family. As we might imagine, intense unconscious anger at the parents did have to be explored. The school phobia cleared up as the boy began to realize that thinking angry thoughts about people would not destroy them.

The initial phase of therapy is a time of reality testing, not only for the therapist but also for the patient. The child may be uncertain about whether he can really trust the therapist. He may fear that this adult will laugh at him, scold him, or reveal his secrets to his parents. For many children, spending two or three hours a week with an adult who shows them undivided attention is such an unusual experience that in its novelty it is both pleasurable and disturbing. They may wonder: Where is the catch? Will it last forever? Or will this new relationship only bring new disappointments?

Important groundwork is laid in the first phase of the new relationship. Issues may vary, and communication may take many forms, depending on the "chemistry" of the personalities of the child and the therapist. There is always a need to achieve some stability of perceptions about one another. For the therapist this means increased diagnostic clarity and a certain "feel" for the child's ways; for the child this means a sufficient feeling of familiarity with "this place and this person" for trust to take root.

Levels of communication

Child therapy is often equated with "play therapy." Indeed, the writings of some clinicians perpetuate the belief that it is *play* that does the *therapy*. (Axline, 1947.) Nothing could be further from the truth. Play in therapy is simply a well-paved and much preferred avenue of communication, particularly for young children. Play in itself does not cure. Play is one of many modes of communication that characterize the relationship between child and therapist, but modes of communication are only one aspect of the complex process of interaction called the therapeutic relationship.

The child must be helped to find ways of communicating his feelings, thoughts, apprehensions, and wishes. The therapist is trained to help the child in expressing feelings, reflecting upon events, and integrating conflicts, all of which take place in the context of the total relationship and all of which are the warp and woof of the fabric of cure.

Play materials vary in the extent to which they are structured. They can range from a set of blocks or a piece of clay, which can be many things, to representational objects like a doll or a toy filling station. Nevertheless, most play materials have the potential of becoming avenues of self-expression. Play often carries an oblique message that the child himself is not aware of and that the therapist then decodes. Sometimes the child is partially aware of the meaning of his play, yet he still prefers to play out what is on his mind rather than say it in words. But quite often children can, and do, talk directly about what they are thinking. The degree to which they do so depends on how much they are used to being listened to and also on what kind of relationship they have with their therapists.

It is best to think of communication between child and therapist as occurring on many levels of explicitness. Words or play can serve either the wish to communicate or the wish to hide from others. Below are several examples of the many levels on which children communicate in therapy and the many modalities of directness that may be involved.

> Seven-year-old Joey said he saw a comic book in which someone was chasing a man into an alley. His mood was somber and his tone lacked luster. He continued to talk about some painters who came to his house to paint the basement. He said he would like

to go and watch them but was not sure he was allowed "down there." The therapist wondered if Joey was not concerned about something that might happen "down there," referring indirectly to Joey's night fears, about which he had not been able to talk as yet. Joey continued to talk about going down into the basement, and the therapist suggested that he really did not have to go down there if he did not want to. The *nightmares* were never mentioned directly, although the communication about *fears* was open and direct.

In this example, communication really takes place on two levels, and play is not involved. The indirect content, however, and the use of metaphor (fear of basement for night fears) lend this example *a quality of play*, of make-believe, in which both patient and therapist participate.

The therapist of a five-year-old girl told her that she was going on vacation. The child asked her to step into a child-sized play store and pretended that she was locking the therapist into the store. She said, "You cry all you want, I don't care!" The therapist stayed in her "prison" and said, "Poor me! Everyone goes away and leaves me, and I have to stay here alone!"

The style of communication here is very much like "play therapy," in the sense that the *play action* carries the burden of the message: "I hate you for leaving me and I want to punish you." The child *used available materials* to help communicate her feelings.

A nine-year-old boy was emerging from his shell of defensive shyness and had begun to express his wish to grow up and be a man. On days when he was feeling particularly good, he always left the therapy hour in an imaginary car which was "parked" outside the door. As he started the imaginary engine, he would say to his therapist, "I hope I don't run out of gas before I get home."

In this case the *play materials* (car, engine) *are a product of the child's imagination.* It does not matter if there really is a car or not. As in the first example, the communication is metaphoric, but here the child imagines the existence of the car and "parks" it outside the therapy room.

Note that in all these examples there is a wish to communicate. Even when the relationship between child and therapist is good, this is not always the case. Children are sometimes afraid that they will not be understood even if they express themselves as clearly as they can. Thus they obscure their message as a form of self-protection. Children may also be afraid that they will be too well understood and may obscure their message for that reason. Most often child therapy involves *conflicts over being understood.* The advantage of using play as a means of communication is that one can "back out" of the communication just as quickly as one got into it; after all, it was only make-believe and didn't *mean* anything anyhow. It is for this reason that play is encouraged in child therapy, though few therapists believe today that play in itself has lasting therapeutic value.

Needless to say, there are many more aspects of communication in therapy with children, including communication through physical symptoms, the use of parents and other adults as messengers to the therapist, and of course variations in therapists' receptivity to messages from children, on whatever level they are sent. The purpose of this discussion has been only to give a brief sample of the enormous variety that exists and, above all, to disabuse the student of the idea that children enter therapy the way adults do: "My problem is that. . . ." Young children are seldom capable of such self-awareness and self-report, and when they can reflect upon themselves it is often a sign of great improvement.

The importance of limits

Every therapist who works with children must give serious thought to his attitude about limiting children's freedom to do and say as they wish. Beginning therapists often have a great deal of difficulty setting limits on the behavior of their patients. It makes them feel mean, uptight, prohibitive, and arbitrary. There are many reasons for this. We all recall, with more or less resentment, the times when our parents put limits on our behavior, when the answer to a dearly held childish wish was a definite "no" and we did not understand. "But *why* can't I do it?" is a phrase that keynotes much of childhood experience. Many a favorite relative, teacher, or adult ally became an idol with clay feet the first time that he said "no." For the therapist identified with the experiences of children, with an investment in seeing children happy, it is very difficult to do now with a patient as was once done to him. It would be easier always to be nice, permissive, and facilitating, and never to say "no" to anything a patient wanted to do.

But even the staunchest nondirective therapists admit that total permissiveness in the therapeutic relationship is not really good therapy. In the words of Frederick Winsor:

> There was an old woman with notions quite new,
> She never told children the things they should do,
> She hoisted the covers up over her head
> When people explained where her theories led.[7]

[7] F. Winsor and M. Perry, *The Space Child's Mother Goose* (New York: Simon and Schuster, 1958), p. 11.

It is easy to define the situations that call for limits without doubt: no one would think of allowing a child to endanger himself physically; no adult would hesitate to stop a child from running into the street, climbing too high, or diving too deep. It is also easy to enumerate those circumstances under which limiting the child would be utter folly: no one would think of stopping a child from playing, talking, drawing, or learning how to do something. Unfortunately, patients put the therapist's convictions to great tests about matters not so easily decided. Perhaps one of the most frequently asked questions by beginners is: "Should I let my patient do this or not?"

Let us consider some of the factors that guide therapists in establishing limits in intensive individual therapy with children. One obvious generalization is that limits have to be set whenever the continuation of the relationship is endangered. This is particularly important in the treatment of delinquent children. For example, the therapist himself might not have strong negative feelings about children stealing apples, candies, or other objects from stores. He might easily consider such behavior symptomatic and feel that there are more important things to take up in therapy than moral issues about property rights. But when repeated stealing creates the danger that the child will be "sent up" as a juvenile offender and subsequently placed in a correctional institution, attempts to limit the stealing (for example, by verbally disapproving of it) become necessary to safeguard the continuation of the therapeutic relationship. One cannot treat a patient who has been locked up in a faraway institution! In such cases, the therapist has to take a clear stand independent of his moral judgment. The message to the child is not, "If you do this, I will think you are bad, because one simply does not steal; it is morally wrong." Rather the message is, "If you do this, they will put you away and then I cannot continue to see you; therefore I am opposed to your stealing and I want you to stop it."

There are, of course, less dramatic forms of behavior that may not result in the child being separated from the therapist but that nevertheless endanger the relationship. Sometimes children become very angry with their therapist and threaten to hit him, kick him, or otherwise abuse him. Again the therapist might not really mind being abused; he might feel that such behavior is understandable and acceptable within limits of physical harm to himself. But after having seriously attacked or abused someone, children do feel guilty. Moreover, guilt in connection with an important person is easily converted into anger toward that person. The guilt of the child can often lead to a termination of therapy, for the child may find it easier to "never come back" than to face up to what he did and to how he feels about it. Often therapists place limits on hitting, swearing, spitting, and other forms of abuse by children not because they condemn such behavior as not "nice" but because they have to protect the child against the excessive feelings of guilt that may ensue from such open hostility.

Perhaps the most commonly encountered situations calling for limits are those in which the child asks for a relaxing of the time structure of the therapy hour. Coming late, leaving early, and staying late are the common forms of innocent requests. "Why can't I stay to finish this drawing?" "Why can't I leave early to catch my favorite television show?" Denying such simple requests makes the therapist feel very cruel. After all, what is another ten minutes? What does it matter if, just once, the child leaves the hour early or late? But every therapist knows how dearly he must pay for such permissiveness. If a child is allowed to shorten or lengthen his session once, why not the next time, and then the next? And there may be a next time when it is not possible to concede to the child's wishes. "Yes, I did let you stay late last time, but today I have to leave myself" appears to be a sensible explanation, but children often experience this as capricious inconsistency and turn bitterly on the therapist, in words or in thought, for being like all other adults—unpredictable and arbitrary. For such reasons, children in intensive therapy are held rather strictly to a previously-agreed-upon schedule. The timing of the hour is an important structure, a contract that if broken often, turns the time set aside for the child into a "rubber hour" whose elasticity can soon become a major problem in the relationship.

There is no form of child therapy without the problem of limits. Total permissiveness is often only in the service of the therapist's need to be well liked, to be seen as a nice guy. The promise of total freedom in the therapy ("Here you may do anything you want to do") is really a kind of seduction, and seduction usually contains seeds of disappointment. At best, total permissiveness in child therapy *appears* to be an avenue leading toward a closer relationship; but at the end of that road is a trap.

When therapists explain to their patients what is acceptable and what is off limits during the therapy hour, they are engaging in "structuring"; that is, they are outlining the basis of the contract. Naturally, there are some clauses in the contract that apply to limits on the therapist's actions as well. Observing confidentiality, being on time for sessions with the child, and apprising him ahead of time of vacations and holidays are some of the important aspects of the relationship that structure (or limit) the therapist's behavior. The general assumption is that trust develops better when both patient and therapist are clear on "what is" and "what can be" done, and that the absence of certain simple rules is tantamount to uncertainty and soon becomes a source of anxiety.

The problem of termination

In psychoanalysis criteria of termination involve judgments about the status of the neurotic conflicts that originally brought the patient into treatment and about the status of his relationship to the analyst. Has the unconscious conflict become conscious? Does the patient have more control over his life? Have major childhood events been thoroughly understood? Has the transference relationship been resolved, and is the patient ready to "let go" of this intense experience? It is clear that the answers to all these questions are matters of judgment and that the subject of termination is complex enough to be a rich topic of discussion among analysts and psychotherapists alike. The intensive therapy of children derives many of its criteria for termination from those of psychoanalysis.[8]

Under ideal circumstances, the treatment of a child ends once the original symptoms have cleared up *and* once the therapist is convinced that the change in the child is solid and is indeed an important *redirection* of the developmental course that at the outset was judged to be pathological. In other words, the therapist who treats children intensively would not be satisfied to know that bed-wetting has stopped or that school grades have improved.[9] He would consider such results important but salutory, insufficient in themselves to indicate termination. He would want some evidence that the changes are "deeper" and that they offer the promise of permanence. It is difficult to state in general terms how such judgments are made. Consider a shy, withdrawn child who during the course of therapy has become increasingly outgoing. Clearly, it is very difficult to decide when, at what point, the change in the child should be seen not as just a "bright-

---

[8] See, for example, S. Freud, "Analysis terminable and interminable," in *Collected Papers,* vol. 5, James Strachey, ed. (New York: Basic Books, 1959). This paper was written quite late in the evolution of psychoanalytic theory (1937).

[9] Compared with behavior modification, intensive psychotherapy places low value on symptom inhibition. Since the main goal of various therapies using the conditioning model (behavior therapy, behavior modification, conditioning therapy, extinction therapy, and so on) is rapid alteration of overt behavior, the disappearance of objectionable symptoms clearly marks the end of treatment. For an excellent discussion of the ethical issues involved in forms of behavior control see P. London, *Behavior Control* (New York: Harper and Row, 1969).

ening up" under the influence of the good relationship with the therapist—as a diminution of shyness because the child now has a friend and feels more supported—but rather as a real change in the child's character that is likely to outlast his relationship with the therapist. In the case of shyness, it is perhaps the difference between accepting an invitation to another child's party and coping with the anxiety of then going there, or between actually wishing to initiate new relationships with children and experiencing only minimal anxiety in doing so. In the case of learning difficulties, the question of termination is often a matter of individual conviction. While most dynamically oriented therapists would agree that improved grades are not sufficient in themselves to indicate termination, they would probably disagree considerably concerning definite, positive criteria for ending therapy. Not only are such judgments based on *unverbalized models for "mental health"* and *convictions about what the quality of the child's life should be;* they are also made against a background of clinical understanding that is as yet unsystematized. Since it is difficult to put unsystematized forms of knowledge into the language of textbooks, students of psychotherapy generally learn about these matters in individual supervision and in other forms of apprenticeship.

Nevertheless, there are several considerations related to termination that can be discussed in general terms, independent of the context of particular clinical situations. For example, do you recall having had a grade-school teacher whom you were very attached to and felt that you could not really be happy without? Do you then remember being separated from that teacher and feeling a great deal of pain about it? And was there ever a time when you had occasion to see that important person later, only to find to your surprise that while you still retained feelings of affection for your teacher somehow you had *outgrown* the relationship? The ideal situation in therapy is somewhat akin to this. There comes a time when the child begins to outgrow the relationship, when he is no longer so intensely attached, when other things in life take over and become much more fascinating than coming for therapy, and when these wishes to "move away" from the therapist no longer have the quality of resistance, anger, and conflict about closeness. When this pertains, therapists say that the "transference relationship" is being resolved; the child can do without the therapist. Ideally, intensive therapy ends only when this shift in the relationship has taken place.

What might stand in the way of such an ideal termination? Life creates situations in which therapy has to be terminated prematurely. The child's parents might move away. The therapist might change jobs. The parents might withdraw the child. This last situation sometimes arises when lines of communication with the parents have not been well established and the parents have *never understood* the goals of therapy. In such instances parents are likely to withdraw the child from therapy once the initial symptoms are removed, and it is often too late to explain to them how little symptom removal can mean.

But there is perhaps no greater reason for interference with ideal termination than the therapist's own ambivalence about it. He might wonder for a long time: Is the child really ready to quit? How can I know? How can anyone know? Of course, in the absence of clear-cut criteria for termination it is easy to delay making a judgment. The therapist might imagine that if only there were definitive research studies on when to end therapy with a child, he would not have so much difficulty making a decision. Such thoughts contain more than a grain of truth, but often they reflect the denial of an important internal reality: the therapist has become attached to the child and cannot allow the child to move away from him! Such are the countertransference problems that often stand in the way of ending a relationship with a child; it is for this reason that no textbook discussion can replace self-knowledge on the part of therapists.

Studies on the problems of termination (Taft, 1933; Ekstein,

1966) have pointed out that this is not just a "technical problem" of treatment—that is, one that lends itself to prescriptions and whose procedural aspects can be taught. It has been suggested that termination contains some of the most universal issues of human relationships. Did anything of value really happen if it did not last forever? Was anything of importance really felt if now it comes to an end? Was anything worth saying really said if everything was not told? Such questions connect the experience of being a therapist to the larger experience of being a human being.

Family therapy

Family therapy involves the entire family group working with one or two family therapists assigned to the treatment. All these people generally meet together. Some family members may, of course, be in individual therapy as well. The assumption behind this approach is that the psychopathology of any one member of a family is determined and kept alive by the problems of the relationships within the family. Mother, father, and children are regarded as parts of a total organic system. Thus in the view of the family therapist, one cannot change any single member of the family without changing the others, or even when one can effect change in an isolated member, the change is likely to be more soundly based if it is done in the setting of the entire family. More specifically, and regarding children, the family therapist believes that maladjusted children are first of all reacting to problems in the family, and that even when one can help the child with some of his problems, as in individual treatment, he might be better helped in family therapy. For example, in dealing with a delinquent child a family therapist would regard the delinquency in large measure as a reaction to intrafamilial problems. Explanations of the more orthodox type may be recognized too. The therapist might view the delinquency as a symbolic cry for help, a symptom of deeply lodged conflicts or of secretly feared inadequacies. But he would believe that faulty family relationships are so primary in the causal network that family therapy should be the treatment of first choice.

The following discussion of family therapy will draw largely on the work of Salvador Minuchin and his colleagues, whose *Families of the Slums* (1967) stands as the most important recent contribution not only to family therapy but also to sophisticated thinking about the psychological problems of the poor. It should be noted, however, that family therapy is by no means restricted either to the poor or to people with special psychological problems. In marriage counseling and the treatment of schizophrenics —for all social class groups—family therapy stands as the one of the most recently discovered methods, enthusiastically received by many clinicians.[10]

The basic assumption underlying family therapy may be succinctly stated as follows:

> Throughout their prolonged experiences with each other, family members have evolved a system of mechanisms for exchanging and negotiating around areas of conflict. As a result of years of accommodation to areas in which there is tension, they have developed systematized ways of organizing, avoiding, manipulating or detouring in situations of stress.
>
> The first goal of the therapist in his attempt to break down these systematized patterns is to watch the family system as it stands so he can roughly identify some areas of stress and the ways family members customarily negotiate around them. However, in our

[10] For an overview see N. Ackerman, "Emergence of family therapy on the present scene," in M. I. Stein (ed.), *Contemporary Psychotherapy* (New York: Free Press, 1961).

view, unobstructed exposure is insufficient for learning about these family systems. Particularly with the disorganized, low socioeconomic family (though not exclusively), it is necessary for the therapist to activate conflict and increase tension as a means of studying the systems. This is necessary because the family's use of accustomed ways of resolving conflict is not well demarcated. (Minuchin *et al.,* 1967, p. 291.)

Just as the body can be viewed as having independent systems of functioning, like the circulatory, respiratory, and digestive systems, so in a family there are processes which may be thought of as separate systems—for example, those pertaining to communication, affectional ties, and roles. Also, just as the body has separate functional subsystems that operate in conjunction with other parts, such as the heart, the liver, and the kidneys, so individual members of the family can function in various subsystems with other members. *Mother* can be thought of as *wife;* she can function in either the parental or the marital subsystem. Mother's favorite *child* can function as *sibling* to another child; he can be part of the parental or the sibling subsystem. The job of the family therapist is to look at the whole and to discern how the family functions, how it communicates, how it resolves conflicts, and how, if at all, it forms suballiances.

As the family therapist (alone or with the co-therapist) discovers the patterns and the ways in which various family processes debilitate the functioning of the entire unit, he clarifies his observations to the family. He has to be a part of the family, but not so much so that he becomes prey to the same faulty communications and distortions that he is trying to change. He must maintain the stance of *participant observer.*

In addition to observing and articulating what is *really* going on in the interactions of family members, the family therapist frequently functions as a model for more effective ways of coping and communicating in the group. He might on occasion ask one member of the family to step into an observation room and view the rest of the family through a one-way mirror. He might film the entire session and then show the family the manner in which various members behave toward one another. (Ackerman, 1961.) The techniques are many and they are all designed to make the therapist serve the entire family unit and to enable the members to see how they affect others, how they create various kinds of impasses, how they attack or fail to defend themselves in the group.

In their studies of slum families, Minuchin and his colleagues were especially impressed with nonproductive communication as a source of deep misunderstanding among family members. For this reason, they developed many techniques for teaching "interpersonal negotiation," to facilitate the "communication traffic":

> Members of the family need not become sophisticated analysts of their own communications, but they should be able to eventually produce some statements which reflect upon their communicational methods. An example of a simple statement which displays growing observational awareness is that of Phyllis Montgomery to her mother [a case discussed at great length], which says, in effect, "I cannot hear you because you always holler at me, so I stop listening." (Minuchin *et al.*, 1967, p. 251.)

Families tend to have their central themes, such as blaming or controlling. Some of these central themes cast people into a rigid role. Families can be helped with the noxious patterns they evolve only by altering the entire family system. For example, children are often placed in the role of scapegoats: if it were not for their misbehavior, school failure, shiftlessness, or delinquency, "everything would be all right"! Scapegoating often results in the internalization of a pathological self-concept.

Through developing and perfecting the techniques of family therapy in their work with the poor, Minuchin and his co-workers have gained increased understanding of how poor families live, what their psychological problems are, and how they typically cope with the pressures of urban life. Minuchin also evolved a typology of family structure that initially was thought to describe only the poor, but that seems to be useful in describing family functioning in all social classes.[11] Two types or styles of functioning emerged particularly clearly: the *disengaged* and the *enmeshed family styles.*

In the disengaged family the members "move as in isolated orbits," as if they were unrelated to one another. There tends to be a long delay in reacting to one another's actions, people do not pay attention to one another, and the children play more in a parallel fashion than together. The mother is likely to feel overwhelmed and depressed. She often complains of illness. She seems unable to control her children. The vacuum left by her unperformed "executive functions" is often filled by a child acting as mother to her younger siblings. She is the "parental child."

The mother is also isolated from the community, and the entire family unit seems to lack anchorage in society. These families tend either to be dropouts from community programs or to have been "taken over" by a social worker. When such a family begins to manipulate social agencies, this may mark the beginning of cohesion; perhaps it is the first sign of a sense of "we."

By contrast, the enmeshed family is characterized by the tight interdependence of its members. They react amply to one another's actions; their verbal interactions escalate quickly. The

[11] I am indebted to Salvador Minuchin for many stimulating discussions about the conceptualization of family styles as described in *Families of the Slums* (New York: Basic Books, 1967) and as subsequently rethought and reformulated by him.

most frequent "engagement maneuver" is the constant controlling behavior of the mother. The development of a "language of affection and concern" is impeded by relentless and vigorous power plays among the children and between the children and the mother. The mother's overwhelming need for control usually excludes the father; even if he is physically present, his psychological role is severely restricted by his wife. Such families tend to view social agencies either as antagonists or as "suckers"; this attitude may reflect the basic feeling of powerlessness among family members that is believed to underlie their constant attempts to control one another.

In the enmeshed family the main currency of interchange between the children and the mother is rebellion. The main aim of therapy is often to make the mother aware of the burden of her power needs in order to enable her to loosen her control over the children.

Other family styles defined by Minuchin arrange themselves along a somewhat different dimension than the disengaged-enmeshed continuum and concern the degree to which parents really function as parents in the psychological sense. For example, in the *nonevolved family style* the parental roles have been abdicated to the grandmother, who functions as parent to the mother as well as to the (grand)children. The *peripheral male* and *juvenile family styles* reflect the structure that may arise when there is no functioning father or when adolescents marry and try to create a family.

The clinical possibilities of family therapy are enormous, but the practice of family therapy is still quite new. Social workers, psychologists, and psychiatrists engage in family therapy, and many psychoanalysts have also become "converted" in their thinking to the view that the family is the patient. Only further research will tell us with what kinds of patients family therapy is more likely to get results than individual therapy. Some forms of illness are more private than others.

Educationally oriented residential treatment

In moving from a discussion of forms of therapy for which children are brought to an office to the kinds for which they are placed in residence, a new set of considerations enters the picture. We must now take into account not only *treatments* (child analysis, family therapy, behavior therapy) but also *programs* and *settings*. Programs take place in or are conducted under the auspices of institutions. They are at least in part publicly financed. The treatment the child receives in such programs—whether it is therapy, education, or both—is never administered by just one person. Therapy is done by the entire milieu.

The description of residential treatment of any kind is thus made more difficult by the very complexity of institutions. Perhaps a comparison with public schools will demonstrate the difficulty of description in this regard. One can compare schools with regard to teacher-pupil ratio, teaching philosophy, and so on. One can also talk about the various and differing goals that schools hold out for their pupils and the policies they have with regard to parents' participation. But clearly even after a very careful description of all these dimensions has been made, one would still not know what happens when all the parts are put together to create an experience. There are *atmospheric aspects of institutions* which are very complex, which convey a total mood, a feeling, a posture toward children. No adequate description of these aspects has ever been formulated, but everyone who has worked in any institution for children "knows" about them.

It makes sense, then, not to talk abstractly about residential treatment for children. It is better to focus on particular programs and to analyze their aims and accomplishments. In the case of individual treatment—the usual once- or twice-a-week "outpatient" therapy—one can talk about treatment methods apart from the setting, but in discussing residential therapy one can never separate the residence from the therapy.

The focus of this discussion will be a new and still somewhat controversial program for emotionally disturbed children known as Project Re-Ed. There are many indications that Project Re-Ed has already become a prototype—several communities have copied the original program, and several more intend to do so. Project Re-Ed not only involves a new approach to treating children; it also calls for a new model for training young people to work with children.

The first Project Re-Ed school was established in 1961 at George Peabody College in Nashville, Tennessee, through the collaborative efforts of the college, the National Institute of Health, and the states of Tennessee and North Carolina. It was stimulated by the widening gap between the needs of emotionally disturbed children and clinical facilities for their cure. Dr. Nicholas Hobbs and his able staff responded to incidence and prevalence figures made public by the biometrics branch of the National Institute of Mental Health; these statistics indicated that the period 1963–1973 would see an increase of 116 percent over the previous decade in the number of children aged ten to fourteen admitted to mental hospitals.

Hobbs and his colleagues became disturbed by this prospect, particularly since they had reason to believe that mental hospitals still regarded children (as most of them today do) as miniature adults and did not understand the special treatment requirements of children and their families. Hobbs believed that even if existing clinical facilities were to redouble their efforts to admit and treat children, such efforts would become shipwrecked simply because of the lack of trained specialists in all fields of mental health. Furthermore, there was good reason to question whether all mental health personnel really needed such sophisticated training as psychologists and psychiatrists receive. Perhaps a whole new way of thinking about therapy was needed, one that was not illness oriented but health oriented, one aimed not at total cure but simply at aiding the child "back on the track" of the larger community and the school. Since there were only about fifty recognized residential treatment centers in the United States in 1961 (there are not many more now) and the cost per child was about $10,000 per year (much more now, in some cases more than $20,000 per year), Hobbs and his colleagues did not have much difficulty convincing fund-dispensing authorities that the time had come to try something new.

By 1969 it was possible not only to create enthusiasm for the continued support of Re-Ed schools but also to clearly communicate the structure, aim, and methods of Re-Ed. Today research is being conducted to demonstrate the degree of improvement that can be expected to take place through Re-Ed. While control group data are still needed, follow-up studies of disturbed children treated through Re-Ed have permitted hopeful conclusions. Parents reported marked improvement in their children's behavior six months after discharge. Teachers reported decreased disruptiveness, increased ability to face difficulties, and increased ability to get along with classmates. A comparison of Metropolitan Achievement Test scores before and after Re-Ed revealed that the insidious "growth in academic gap between Re-Ed children and their peers was arrested." (Weinstein, 1969, p. 71.) Should the study of a control group of disturbed children reveal that the passage of time alone cannot account for these improvements, all this evidence will of course become more conclusive.

In the meantime, the concepts of Re-Ed are evolving into a distinct point of view about how to help mentally ill children. The basic assumption is that such youngsters should not be "sent away," as they often are; rather they should be treated close to the community, in its mainstream, as it were. All Re-Ed schools are residential centers, but they are located near public transportation lines so that parents can come and go and children can visit their homes and return easily. This puts contact with families on a flexible basis. (In state hospitals it is extremely difficult to obtain permission for a child to go home for the weekend.)

The Re-Ed concept of ecological planning calls for intensive camp experiences in which children can learn to master real-life difficulties and feel themselves competent to perform such basic tasks as preparing food and making shelter. Special abilities of children in the academic areas are identified and highlighted to provide them with a feeling of success and competence, even if this sense of competence is limited at the outset.

Several techniques of Re-Ed are novel in that they have not been used with disturbed children in quite the same way. Survival camping is seen as very important in giving boys and girls a feeling of personal effectiveness through the competent use of the body. There is a clearly stated goal that each child should have some experience of *joy* each day, that something should happen to him—be it a trip, a project, or an event—that will cause him to look forward to *this day* and that will take him away from the ordinary and out of his despair. Not inconsistent with this is the belief that it is very important for each child to be alone part of the day, to be allowed to withdraw and be only with himself.

In addition to emphasizing the importance of setting—the camp, the school, the "places" in which children learn to live— Re-Ed focuses on the role of teacher counselors. The idea of *éducateurs* in small residential schools was originated by Robert Lafon and Henri Joubel of France. But the role of Re-Ed counselors was also shaped by Campbell Loughmiller's ideas on camping for disturbed boys, as well as by the model provided by Peace Corps workers all over the world. The teacher counselor at Re-Ed has psychiatrists and psychologists available for consultation. But the counselor is given primary responsibility to plan the activities of small groups of children and to serve as liaison between these youngsters and their home and school. (Hobbs, 1969.)

What are some of the principles that guide those who plan

the activities of the children? Because Re-Ed was developed not out of a particular personality theory but out of an acute social need, the list of guiding principles is anything but a theoretician's delight. Rather it is a set of beliefs that some ways of thinking about children are not profitable or practical, while others serve the children better now, when they are disturbed. There is, then, little attempt at formulating a cohesive theory of mental illness or anything close to it. Critics of Re-Ed often point to this as a shortcoming.

In 1964 Hobbs described Re-Ed as having several strong biases. One is a bias in favor of thinking about the child not as sick but as having acquired bad habits:

> We assume that he has learned to construe the world in such a way that his world must reject him, and that he has acquired specific ways of coping that are immediately rewarding but ultimately defeating. The task of re-education is to help the child learn new and more effective ways of construing himself and his world and to learn habits that lead to more effective functioning. (Hobbs, 1964, p. 3.)

Another strong bias in Re-Ed thinking is a deliberate avoidance of "preoccupation with intrapsychic processes." Instead, there is a preoccupation with the ecology of the child, his relationship to the larger system that contains him, his school, and his family. The statement of this belief recognizes its possible limitations regarding "depth of cure":

> We assume that life is more healing than we are, and that our intervention is an emergency measure, that our goal is not the complete remaking of a child. What we try to do is to get the child, the family, the school, and the community just enough above the threshold of the requirements of each from the other, so that the

whole system has a just-significant margin of probable success over probable failure. . . . It is possible for a system to work without the necessity of any intrapsychic change in the child at all. (Hobbs, 1964, p. 4.)

Because of such biases, Re-Ed does not use diagnostic terms in dealing with children; nor do Re-Ed teachers engage in therapy in the conventional sense. While there is a recognition that phenomena of therapy (transference, regression, counter-transference) do occur in working with children in Re-Ed settings, there is no special interest in "exploiting" the treatment potentials of these phenomena. Yet we may wonder whether this is simply a rejection of traditional categories and terms. Re-Ed places strong emphasis on helping children to develop trust in the adults who care for them, on obtaining the children's cooperation in *giving up* objectionable behavior (symptoms), and on teaching them to adhere to middle class standards of behavior. It is hard for this writer to think of such goals out of the context of the child's relationship with the counselor. We may not call this therapy, and we may not call it transference. And for some purposes this may not matter at all. What the Re-Ed staff seems deeply to recognize is the power of human ties.

References

Ackerman, N. "Emergence of family therapy on the present scene." In M. I. Stein, ed., *Contemporary Psychotherapy*. New York: Free Press, 1961.

American Psychological Association. *Ethical Standards of Psychologists*. Washington, D.C.: American Psychological Association, 1953.

Ariès, P. *Centuries of Childhood*. New York: Alfred A. Knopf, 1962.

Axline, V. *Play Therapy.** Boston: Houghton Mifflin, 1947.

Bettelheim, B. *The Empty Fortress*. New York: Free Press, 1967.

Binet, A. *Les idées modernes sur les enfants.** Paris: Flammarion, 1911.

Bowlby, J. *Attachment*. New York: Basic Books, 1969.

———. *Maternal Care and Mental Health.** New York: Schocken Books, 1967. Originally published in 1951 by the World Health Organization.

Browning, R. M., and D. O. Stover. *Behavior Modification in Child Treatment*. Chicago: Aldine, 1971.

* Available in paperback.

REFERENCES

Des Lauriers, A. M. *The Experience of Reality in Childhood Schizophrenia.* New York: International Universities Press, 1962.

Dittmann, L. L., ed. *Early Child Care.* New York: Atherton Press, 1968.

Engel, M. "On the psychological testing of borderline children." *AMA Archives of General Psychiatry,* 8 (1963), 426–34.

———. "Children who work." *AMA Archives of General Psychiatry,* 17 (1967), 291–97.

———. "Dilemmas of classification and diagnosis." *Journal of Special Education,* 3 (1969), 231–39.

Ekstein, R. *Children of Time, Space, Action, and Impulse.* New York: Appleton-Century-Crofts, 1966.

Fenichel, O. *The Psychoanalytic Theory of Neuroses.* New York: W. W. Norton, 1945.

Freud, A. *Psychoanalytical Treatment of Children.* London: Imago, 1946.

———. *The Ego and the Mechanisms of Defense.* New York: International Universities Press, 1960.

———. *Normality and Pathology of Childhood.* New York: International Universities Press, 1965.

———. "A short history of child analysis." In *The Psychoanalytic Study of the Child,* vol. 21. New York: International Universities Press, 1966.

Freud, S. "Analysis of a phobia in a five-year-old-boy." In *Collected Papers,* vol. 3, Ernest Jones, ed., Alix and James Strachey, trans. New York: Basic Books, 1959.

———. "Analysis terminable and interminable." In *Collected Papers,* vol. 5, James Strachey, ed. New York: Basic Books, 1959.

Glidewell, J. C. "The prevalence of maladjustment in elementary schools." Mimeographed report prepared for the Joint Commission on Mental Health of Children, December 1967.

Golden, M., and W. Bridger. "A refutation of Jensen's position on intelligence, race, social class, and heredity." *Mental Hygiene,* 53 (1969), 648–53.

REFERENCES

Goldfarb, W. *Childhood Schizophrenia.* Cambridge, Mass.: Harvard University Press, 1961.

————, Mintz, I., and K. W. Stroock. *A Time to Heal.* New York: International Universities Press, 1969.

Group for the Advancement of Psychiatry. *Psychological Disorders in Childhood: Theoretical Considerations and a Proposed Classification.** New York: Group for the Advancement of Psychiatry, 1966.

Hammer, M. M., and A. M. Kaplan. *The Practice of Psychotherapy with Children.* Homewood, Ill.: Dorsey Press, 1967.

Haworth, M. *Child Psychotherapy.* New York: Basic Books, 1964.

Heinicke, C., and I. Westheimer. *Brief Separations.* New York: International Universities Press, 1969.

Hinde, R. A. *Animal Behaviour, A Synthesis of Ethology and Comparative Psychology.* New York: McGraw-Hill, 1966.

Hobbs, N. "The process of re-education." Paper delivered at the first annual workshop for the staff of Project Re-Ed, Gatlinburg, Tennessee, 1964. Mimeographed.

————. *Project Re-Ed, New Concepts for Helping Emotionally Disturbed Children.* Brochure. Nashville, Tenn.: George Peabody College, 1969.

Jenkins, R. L., and J. O. Cole. *Diagnostic Classification in Child Psychiatry,* Psychiatric Research Report No. 18. Washington, D.C.: American Psychiatric Association, 1964.

Joint Commission on Mental Health of Children. *Crisis in Child Mental Health.* New York: Harper and Row, 1970.

Kaplan, A. *The Conduct of Inquiry.* San Francisco: Chandler, 1964.

Kessler, J. W. *Psychopathology of Childhood.* Englewood Cliffs, N.J.: Prentice-Hall, 1966.

London, P. *Behavior Control.* New York: Harper and Row, 1969.

Mahler, M. S. *On Human Symbiosis and the Vicissitudes of Individuation.* New York: International Universities Press, 1968.

Mead, M., and M. Wolfenstein, eds. *Childhood in Contemporary Cultures.** Chicago: University of Chicago Press, 1963.

Minuchin, S., *et al. Families of the Slums.* New York: Basic Books, 1967.

National Clearing House for Mental Health Information. *The National Institute of Mental Health,** Information Publication No. 5027. Washington, D.C.: U.S. Government Printing Office, 1970.

Prugh, D. Remarks quoted in "Psychiatrists clarify Joint Commission report on children." *Frontiers of Hospital Psychiatry,* 7 (1970), 1–11.

Rogers, C. *Client-Centered Therapy.* Boston: Houghton Mifflin, 1951.

Rosen, B. M., Bahn, A. K., and M. Kramer. "Demographic and diagnostic characteristics of psychiatric clinic outpatients in the U.S.A., 1961." *American Journal of Orthopsychiatry,* 34 (1964), 455–68.

Shakow, D., and D. Rapaport. *The Influence of Freud on American Psychology.** New York: International Universities Press, 1964.

Shapiro, D. *Neurotic Styles.* New York: Basic Books, 1965.

Sherwood, M. *The Logic of Explanation in Psychoanalysis.* New York: Academic Press, 1969.

Simpson, G. G. *Principles of Animal Taxonomy.* New York: Columbia University Press, 1961.

Sluckin, W. *Imprinting and Early Learning.** Chicago: Aldine, 1965.

Snow, C. P. *Science and Government.* Cambridge, Mass.: Harvard University Press, 1961.

Sugarman, J. M. "Research, evaluation, and public policy." *Child Development,* 41 (1970), 263–66.

Szasz, T. S. "The problem of psychiatric nosology." *American Journal of Psychiatry,* 114 (1957), 405–13.

Taft, J. *The Dynamics of Therapy in a Controlled Relationship.* New York: Macmillan, 1933.

Waelder, R. *Basic Theory of Psychoanalysis.* New York: International Universities Press, 1960.

Warren Commission. *Report of the Warren Commission on the Assassination of President John F. Kennedy.** New York: Bantam Books, 1964.

Weinstein, L. "Project Re-Ed schools for emotionally disturbed children: effectiveness as viewed by referring agencies, parents, and teachers." *Exceptional Children, 35* (1969), 703–11.

Whiting, B. B., ed. *Six Cultures—Studies of Child Rearing.* New York: John Wiley and Sons, 1963.

Winsor, F., and M. Perry. *The Space Child's Mother Goose.* New York: Simon and Schuster, 1958.

Wolins, M. "Child care in cross-cultural perspective." Mimeographed. Berkeley: University of California, Department of Social Welfare, 1969.

Yarrow, L. J. "Maternal deprivation: toward an empirical and conceptual evaluation." *Psychological Bulletin, 58* (1961), 459–90.

Zigler, E., and L. Philips. "Psychiatric diagnosis: a critique." *Journal of Abnormal Social Psychology, 63* (1961), 607–18.

Suggested Readings

Infancy

Brazelton, T. B. *Infants and Mothers—Differences in Development.* New York: Delacorte Press, 1969.

Chess, S., and A. Thomas, eds. *Annual Progress in Child Psychiatry and Child Development.* New York: Brunner Mazel, 1968, 1969, 1970.

Foss, B. M., ed. *Determinants of Infant Behaviour,* vols. 1–4. London: Methuen, 1961–1969.

Hellmuth, J., ed. *Exceptional Infant.* Vol. 1, *The Normal Infant.* Seattle: Special Child Publications, 1967. Vol. 2, *Studies in Abnormalities.* New York: Brunner Mazel, 1971.

Seen, M. J. E., and C. Hartford. *The Firstborn.* Cambridge, Mass.: Harvard University Press, 1968.

Spitz, R. *The First Year of Life.* New York: International Universities Press, 1965.

* Available in paperback.

The middle years of childhood

Anthony, J. E., and T. Benedek. *Parenthood, Its Psychology and Psychopathology.* Boston: Little Brown, 1970.

Clarizio, H. F., and G. F. McCoy. *Behavior Disorders in School-Age Children.* Scranton, Pa.: Chandler, 1970.

Gardner, R. W., and A. Moriarty. *Personality Development at Preadolescence.* Seattle: University of Washington Press, 1968.

Millar, S. *The Psychology of Play.* Baltimore: Penguin Books, 1968.

Murphy, L. B. *The Widening World of Childhood.* New York: Basic Books, 1962.

Adolescence

Aichhorn, A. *Wayward Youth.* New York: Meridian Books, 1960.

Hirsch, E. A. *The Troubled Adolescent as He Emerges on Psychological Tests.* New York: International Universities Press, 1970.

Jacobs, J. *Adolescent Suicide.* New York: John Wiley and Sons, 1971.

Parker, B. *My Language Is Me.* New York: Basic Books, 1962.

Plath, S. *The Bell Jar.* New York: Harper and Row, 1971.

Children in groups

Bettelheim, B. *The Children of the Dream.* New York: Macmillan, 1969.

Furman, R. A., and A. Katan. *The Therapeutic Nursery School.* New York: International Universities Press, 1969.

Rabin, A. L. *Growing Up in the Kibbutz.* New York: Springer, 1965.

Redl, F. *When We Deal with Children.* New York: Free Press, 1966.

Poverty and racism

Agee, J., and W. Evans. *Let Us Now Praise Famous Men*. Boston: Houghton Mifflin, 1960.

Allen, V. L., ed. *Psychological Factors in Poverty*. Chicago: Markham, 1970.

Coles, R. *Children of Crisis*. Boston: Little Brown, 1964.

Deutsch, M., *et al. The Disadvantaged Child*. New York: Basic Books, 1967.

Dohrenwend, B. P., and B. S. Dohrenwend. *Social Status and Psychological Disorder*. New York: John Wiley and Sons, 1969.

Kozol, J. *Death at an Early Age.** New York: Bantam Books, 1967.

Williams, F. *Language and Poverty*. Chicago: Markham, 1970.

Special handicaps

Furth, H. G. *Thinking Without Language—Psychological Implications of Deafness*. New York: Free Press, 1966.

Money, J., ed. *The Disabled Reader—Education of the Dyslexic Child*. Baltimore: Johns Hopkins Press, 1966.

Strauss, A. A., and N. Kephart. *Psychopathology and Education of the Brain-Injured Child,* vol. 1. New York: Grune and Stratton, 1965.

————, and L. E. Lehtinen. *Psychopathology and Education of the Brain-Injured Child,* vol. 2. New York: Grune and Stratton, 1965.

Wender, P. H. *Minimal Brain Dysfunction in Children*. New York: John Wiley and Sons, 1971.

The course of therapy: first-person accounts

Baruch, D. *One Litle Boy*. New York: Julian Press, 1952.

Green, H. *I Never Promised You a Rose Garden.** New York: Signet Books, 1964.

Parker, B. *My Language Is Me*. New York: Basic Books, 1962.

Theoretical considerations in child psychology

London, P. *Behavior Control.** New York: Harper and Row, 1969.
Lorenz, K. *On Aggression.* New York: Harcourt Brace Jovanovich, 1963.
Lovaas, O. I. "A behavior therapy approach to the treatment of childhood schizophrenia." In J. Hill, ed., *Minnesota Symposium on Child Psychiatry.* Minneapolis: University of Minnesota Press, 1967.
Munroe, R. *School of Psychoanalytic Thought.* New York: Dryden Press, 1955.
Wolff, P. H. *The Developmental Theories of Jean Piaget and Psychoanalysis.** New York: International Universities Press, 1960.

Genetics

Rosenthal, D. *Genetics of Psychopathology.** New York: McGraw-Hill, 1971.

Childhood in autobiography

Brown, C. *Manchild in the Promised Land.** New York: Signet Books, 1965.
Cohen, M. R. *A Dreamer's Journey.* New York: Free Press, 1948.
Gide, A. *If It Die . . . An Autobiography.** Translated by Dorothy Bussy. New York: Vintage Books, 1935.
Gorki, M. *Childhood.* Translated by Margaret Wettlin; translation revised by Jessie Coulson. London: Oxford University Press, 1961.
Proust, M. *Swann's Way.* Translated by C. Scott Moncrieff. New York: Macmillan, 1957.
Russell, B. *Autobiography of Bertrand Russell.* Boston: Little Brown, 1967.

Index

INDEX

Joint Commission on Mental Health of Children, 18, 25n, 29–32, 57, 71n
Joubel, Henri, 164
Juvenile family, 160

Kanner, Leo, 88
Kaplan, A., 95n
Kaplan, A. M., 142n
Kenya, 57
Kessler, J. W., 71n
Kibbutzim, 58–59
Kinderdorf, 58–59
King, William, 48n
Kraepelin, Emil, 66–67
Kramer, M., 35
Kris, Marianne, 135

Lafon, Robert, 164
Lansburgh, Mrs. Richard, 14–15
Learning theory, 97
Legal Aid Society, 12–13
Life magazine, 14
Lincoln-Oseretsky Test, 87
Lindemann, F. A., 19
Little Hans, psychoanalysis of, 132–35
London, P., 152n
Lorenz, K., 79
Loughmiller, Campbell, 164
Love object, anxiety over loss of, 98

Mahler, Margaret, 88–94, 135
Maladjustment, among schoolchildren, 33–38
Marasmus, 45
Martin, John B., 15
Mass media, public information and, 11–17
Masturbation, 44, 99–100
Maternal associations, 44
Maternity care, 26–28
Mead, Margaret, 42n, 43–46
Melancholy, mild chronic, 104
Mental disorders, incidence of, 16

Mental hospitals, admissions to, 162
Mexico, 57
Middle Ages, 40
Mintz, I., 83
Minuchin, Salvador, 156–60
Moralism, religious, 41, 44–45
Moral necessity, in obsessive-compulsive neurosis, 122
Mothers: role in child-raising, 42–43, 48–60; schizophrenogenic, 92–93; separation of child from natural, 52–60; working, 51, 56–57
Mortality, infant, 27
Motility, 75
Motivation, in schizophrenia, 85
Multiple or shared caretaking, 22, 55–60
Murray, Henry A., 107
Mutism, 76

National Clearing House for Mental Health Information, 16n
National Institute of Health, 162
National Institute of Mental Health, 36, 55, 162
"Nature-nurture" controversy, and schizophrenia, 90
Nechin, Herbert, 48n
Neglect and abuse of children, 11–13
Neurosis. *See* Psychoneurosis, childhood
Neurotic Styles (Shapiro), 119–23
New York City, 12–15
New York Times, 11–14, 15n
Nondirective therapy, 1–29, 127
Noninvolved family, 160

Obsessive-compulsive neurosis, 105–24; moral necessity in, 122; reality in, 122–23; rigidity in, 119–20; will and volition in, 120–21
Organicity, tests of, 86–87
Orthogenic School (University of Chicago), 77ff.

A 2
B 3
C 4
D 5
E 6
F 7
G 8
H 9
I 0
J 1